Complete Guide
to Prevention
and Treatment of
Athletic Injuries

Complete Guide to Prevention and Treatment of Athletic Injuries

B. J. BROWN

PARKER PUBLISHING COMPANY, INC.
West Nyack, N.Y.

© 1972 *by*

Parker Publishing Company, Inc.
West Nyack, N.Y.

Library of Congress Cataloging in Publication Data

```
Brown, B    J    (date)
   Complete guide to prevention and treatment of
athletic injuries.

   1.  Sports--Accidents and injuries.  I.  Title:
[DNLM:  1.  Athletic injuries--Prevention and control.
2.  Athletic injuries--Therapy.  QT 260 B877c  1972]
RD131.B73          617'.1027          72-4868
ISBN 0-13-160275-6
```

Printed in the United States of America

THIS BOOK IS DEDICATED TO
Barbara and Brandon
Mother and Daddy
Mama Bard
Aunt Skeet
George and B. J.

Acknowledgements

The following people in my opinion helped make this book a reality:

The late Kenneth Knox, Athletic Director, Southeast Missouri State College, who made it possible for me to obtain a college education and who started me in athletic training.

J. Hugh May, formerly Superintendent of Schools, East Prairie, Missouri, who encouraged me to participate in athletics and who assisted me in getting into college.

Ray Melton, Superintendent of Schools, East Prairie, Missouri, who taught me basketball and how to be a gentleman on and off the athletic field of play.

Homer Rice, Athletic Director, University of North Carolina, and Ray Callahan, Head Football Coach, University of Cincinnati, who offered numerous suggestions relative to the training room and who have demonstrated that "good guys" can finish first.

Chris Patrick, Athletic Trainer, University of Florida, who provided material for the completion of the book.

Adolph F. Rupp, Head Basketball Coach, University of Kentucky, who initiated me into big time athletics, and who taught me how to win and lose gracefully and to act responsibly under great mental and physical stress.

Robert Spackman, Athletic Trainer, Southern Illinois University, who taught me most of what I know about athletic training.

Eddie Ferrell, Football Trainer, and Ed Motley, Basketball Trainer, Virginia Tech, who gave generously of their time and facilities so that illustrations could be prepared.

Richard Amsden, Richard Marquez, Cary Lee Nichols, Larry Smith, and John Sprenkle, who posed for the photographs.

Dr. Herbert Sorenson, a former college teacher of mine, who always encouraged me to publish my ideas.

How This Book Will Help You

This book contains a systematic approach to causes, prevention, treatment and rehabilitation of athletic injuries. It has been written to provide answers to the many questions posed while I was an athletic trainer at Southeast Missouri State College, Southern Illinois University and the University of Kentucky.

Because of these frequent inquiries from schools, colleges, and youth leagues, it became apparent that there was a general lack of athletic training knowledge in some of these programs provided by these groups. Consequently, many athletes were in danger of having promising careers ended because of improperly handled injuries.

Since injuries do and will continually occur, I have written this book primarily for the coach who must be his own trainer or who must supervise the injury care program delegated to the student trainers who have limited expertise in athletic training, but it will prove equally useful for the director of youth league sports programs who always works within a limited budget and the college instructor who teaches a basic athletic training course to prospective physical education teachers and coaches.

To meet the needs of these three groups, the book has been written and organized to provide a fast, efficient method for returning an athlete to good health. Therefore, the user of this book will

1. not lose an important contest because of an injury to a valuable athlete
2. have his players so mentally and physically prepared they

will be able to meet the demand for maximum strength and conditioning always needed in the later stages of a contest

3. avoid adverse public reaction to his program because of unnecessary and poorly handled injuries

4. gain the confidence of educators when they realize that the coach is vitally concerned with the athlete's total welfare

5. save the school and the athletic program money by keeping minor injuries from developing into major problems

6. send from his school athletes who are more aware of the preventive aspects of sports medicine and of the great contributions athletics could make to the total health of all people.

JOE BROWN

Contents

1

Developing a Medical Policy

NEED FOR ATHLETIC TRAINING

Athletic training is a systematic approach to causes, prevention, treatment, and rehabilitation of athletic injuries. It is made important by the complexity of modern sports and the large number of participants engaged in athletics at all age levels.

The magnitude of modern sports have resulted in the development of detailed organizational programs to handle any detrimental situation that might arise. Nevertheless, some of these programs often overlook one of the most important contributors to any successful team—the protection of the student-athlete's physical welfare.

The welfare of athletes in relation to winning teams grows in stature as more emphasis is placed on the win-loss record. Schools with this emphasis often feel that the coach, not the available material, is the primary reason for the great seasons. However, progressive schools do not rely wholly upon the coach; they advocate essential conditioning and protection to forestall the possibilities of injury to their student-athletes who enter athletic competition.

Since the outcome of athletic events is often affected by injuries, a day hardly passes without the sports pages carrying stories about injuries to various players. Many of these stories are possible exaggerations designed to make opponents overconfident of victory, but regardless of any disproportionate publicity, there are sometimes unnecessary complications from sports injuries, especially in junior and senior high school.

Therefore, thorough measures for injury prevention must be followed throughout the sports season so that athletes are capable of meeting the demand for maximum strength and condition and so that adverse public reaction can be prevented. You need the confidence of the public in order to promote a successful athletic program, and your understanding of athletic training can be helpful in assuring this vital public confidence.

The first step in preparing this foundation of public confidence includes, besides a personal knowledge of anatomy, kinesiology, physiology, and psychology, a method of organization. This organizational plan includes (a) a medical and insurance policy, (b) a training room design, and (c) a procedure for testing, treating and rehabilitating athletic injuries.

MEDICAL POLICY

A well-organized and administered medical policy will promote confidence in the athletic program, and you must have this policy well-established, especially when entering a new school system. Ideally, the medical policy includes (a) a professionally qualified and athletically oriented physician, (b) an insurance program with a written policy regarding financial responsibility for athletic injuries and (c) a written injury protection and care policy for practice and games.

Team Physician

The team physician is one of the most important persons associated with the athletic program; especially since his diagnosis will often affect the athlete's health and perhaps the season's outcome. He, therefore, must be chosen on the basis of his medical knowledge of athletic injuries and his ability to get along with young people. Never should the team physician be selected because of political pressure, but he must be chosen on the basis of his professional qualifications and the following vital considerations.

1. He should be a professionally qualified general practitioner or orthopedist who has participated in athletics or who at least understands and believes in the athletic program. He should know the inherent values of athletics and understand the social phenomenon of competitive sports, and he should not publicly belittle any segment of the over-all athletic program.

2. He should have an established practice so that he can attend games and quite ideally practice sessions. If he is unable to attend, he should be well-enough established to obtain a suitable substitute, and he should also be available for emergencies at any time, day or night.

3. He should recognize the worth of each individual athlete, and he must maintain a relationship of friendliness with the athletes so that he can promote confidence and cooperation in the athletic program.

4. He should be a man whom you respect and trust, and before he assists in setting up an athletic program, he should also understand that athletic injuries often require methods of treatment and rehabilitation different from those used for other injuries.

5. He should be able to gain the parents' respect and to help them understand the importance of training and conditioning in injury prevention. He should be willing to help you gain parental support and cooperation in curfews and other rules which help develop a successful athletic program.

6. He should be able to judge an injury solely on its medical merits, withstanding parental concern, emotional involvement, and undue pessimism in both the athlete who is hesitant to return to participation and the one who is withheld from participation.

Insurance Program

Another important aspect of the medical policy is the provision for appropriate insurance coverage for all those participating in the athletic program. This coverage is an excellent method of protecting and helping you as well as the team physician, the athlete, and the school. It is also important that each have a written copy of the policy regarding financial responsibility for athletic injuries. This policy must describe in detail the type of insurance program available for payment of hospital and medical care and should be based on the following criteria.

1. It must provide ways of meeting all the financial responsibilities brought about by an athletic injury, and ideally its provisions should provide for immediate diagnostic and medical attention with X rays, transportation, and hospitalization.
2. It must be adaptable to local conditions and needs.
3. It must cover all athletes who participate in the athletic program.
4. It must be economical for both the parent and the school.
5. It must, in case of tight financial situations, be flexible enough to be integrated with the parents' insurance policies.

Practice and Game Policy

The third important factor for a successful medical policy is an organizational guide for practices and games. This guide includes the following provisions:

1. Each athlete should be given a thorough pre-season physical examination including eyes, ears, nose, teeth, heart, lungs, genitals, joints and muscles. A complete personal history of childhood diseases and respiratory difficulties should also be included (Appendix 1 contains a form for this purpose). When possible there should be complete laboratory tests, inoculations for flu, tetanus, and polio, and X rays of chest and back. The team physician gives the examination when all athletes can participate and records the results at that time. If parents insist, family physicians may assist in the physical examination.
2. Accurate records of physical examinations (Appendix 2 contains a form for this purpose) and injuries must be kept. These records enable you to ascertain the athletes who will need corrective work. It will also enable you to determine the cause of some injuries and be better prepared for prevention of further injury. The keeping of accurate records may also be helpful should a liability suit be brought against you or the school.
3. Parents' cooperation in the athletic training program can be assured by having them check on the daily condition of their sons and report any deviation from normal health such as boils, minor cuts, and colds.
4. Athletes must be instructed to weigh before and after practice. Excessive loss or gain of weight should be investigated immediately. It is good to have a student trainer supervise the weighing-in procedure to assure recording of weight. When immediate weight loss

is equal to 5 per cent of the athlete's normal weight, he must be sent to the team physician for a checkup.

5. Provisions for the best available practice and game equipment is a must, and this equipment must be clean and in good repair.

6. Athletes must be instructed in proper fundamentals. This essential instruction has a double purpose of achieving the most effective execution of the skill and of further protecting athletes from disabling injuries.

7. Squad practice of fundamentals should be arranged so that there is adequate room for participants to carry out their tasks without endangering other squad members. Whenever groups are placed too close together, there is danger of collisions which can cause serious injuries.

8. Competent officials must be employed. A good measure of excellence finds officials who are highly skilled in the technical phase of officiating and who recognize their responsibilities regarding the prevention of injuries.

9. Student trainers should be appointed to help in the care and treatment of athletic injuries, and they should be instructed in the basic first-aid for athletic injuries. It is advisable to enroll each of your student trainers in the Student Trainer's Course (Appendix 3 contains an application form) provided by the Cramer Chemical Company, Gardner, Kansas. Additionally, you should request that Cramer's send you the monthly *First Aider* and the Bike Sales Division of the Kendall Company, Chicago, Illinois, send you *Bike Sports Trails*.

10. A stretcher as well as a training kit must be provided for every practice and game. The training kit includes the following:

Airway	Germicide
Alcohol	Hand Mirror
Ammonia Capsules	Oral Screw
Analgesic Balm	Rosin
Aspirin	Salt Tablets
Antiseptics	Skin Toughener
Band-aides	Sponge Rubber
Bandage Rolls	Sterile Pads
Charley Horse wraps	Tape
Chemical Ice	Teeth Protectors
Cotton Tipped Applicators	Telfa Pads
Elastic Wraps	Tongue Depressors
Foot and Body Powder	Tongue Forceps

11. A responsible individual should be at each practice and game with the following equipment on his person:

Airway   Sterile Gauze Pads
Ammonia Capsules   Tape Scissors
Band-aides   Tongue Depressors
Oral Screw   Tongue Forceps
Roll of Tape

12. A suitable area for treatment and rehabilitation of injuries should be furnished with basic athletic training supplies and equipment. Appendix 4 gives an example of what supplies are essential for schools with small, moderate, or large budgets. The needed supplies will vary from school to school because of the emphasis placed on the protective measures to be taken. For example, coaches who require that all athletes' ankles be taped or wrapped will need more tape or wraps than a school which does not require taping or wrapping as a protective measure. A more detailed listing of the training room needs is contained in Chapter 2.

2

Building and Renovating the Training Room

The responsibility for the training of your athletes includes setting aside a place for the immediate and continued care of any occurring injury. However, the extra expense involved in providing a specific place for injury care is sometimes opposed by the school administration as being too costly. To meet such opposition, you must be able to describe basic specifications for the training room and tell why it is essential to your injury care program.

Authorities generally agree that the ideal training room is a place specifically set aside for injury care. It has good lighting and ventilation, a constant temperature range of 72 to 78 degrees, light-colored walls, ceilings and floors, and electrical outlets located three to four feet from the floor and spaced at six to eight feet intervals. It is near the dressing room, but not part of it nor is it to be used as a passageway to the dressing room or showers.

Many schools, however, are not endowed with the money or facilities for an ideal training room, and in a majority of cases, you will have to promote the need for a training room. This promotion includes a well-organized plan of action which outlines why the training room is essential to injury care. You will find the following basic points helpful in formulating a plan of action.

1. Many minor injuries often are not reported immediately because

there is no one person to whom they must be reported. The procedure is further complicated by the athlete's apparent reluctance to be treated for these so called minor injuries in the presence of his teammates and the difficulty of giving minor injuries proper attention during the confusion of dressing or undressing.

2. Maintaining a sanitary and comparatively private environment is generally helpful for treatment of athletic injuries. Because of this need from both a practical and psychological point of view, because of the increased public attention given to the athletic injury problem, and because of the need for maintaining the strength of the athletic team, schools have been giving more attention to adequate measures for the protection of the athlete's welfare. The physical presence of training facilities shows the school's and the athletic department's interest in the protection of the athlete's health.

3. A properly fitted training room must be a part of every athletic program, and its cost is minimal compared with monies spent for uniforms and other equipment.

LOCATION

Because many high schools often do not have a separate room set aside for injury care, you may find yourself lacking adequate space and thus must work with whatever space is available. The first thing to look for is a storage or other room which could be converted into a training room, and if there is no such available place, a part of the dressing room can be partitioned and set aside for injury care. You might also cooperate with the school health clinic (department) to provide an area for a health clinic during school hours and a training room for athletic use after school hours, or else the physical education department and athletic department might cooperate to provide athletic training therapy equipment which is jointly used by the physical education department, health department and athletic department.

In locating the training room, space for working and traffic flow is of vital importance. The following requirements for location should be followed as closely as possible; however, if it is not feasible to meet any of these criteria, you must not let this keep you from providing a separate room for injury care.

Ideally, the training room is (a) near the playing area, (b) close to the dressing room and away from shower rooms, (c) close to water and drainage, (d) provided with good lighting, (e) provided with clean facilities, (f) provided with ventilation, (g) easily accessible, and (h) provided with heat.

After the training room area has been located, design it for efficient service for several athletes at one time. This will help eliminate the problems which might throw you off schedule. To further facilitate the elimination of time consuming problems, equipment must be practical and not contribute to the possibility of further injury. It should be designed to save unnecessary footsteps and to provide a completely unhampered and uncomplicated traffic lane. Equipment of a sensitive nature must not be near the traffic lane, and mountable electrical equipment should be easily accessible.

EQUIPMENT

Another important factor in the training room design is equipment which may be either purchased from a sporting goods store or made in the school's vocational training shop.

Heat Lamp

A heat lamp for providing dry heat is a must. If it is not possible to secure a heat lamp, a heating pad is a good substitute. The heat lamp may also be inexpensively constructed from metal tubing, light reflector, electrical wire, and bulbs.

Refrigerator

The refrigerator is necessary for maintenance of an adequate supply of ice for use in treating injuries. A used refrigerator may be purchased in any locality at a reasonable price; just keep in mind that the main feature of this refrigerator is its capacity for making and keeping ice. It is also useful for storing ice bags and cold water.

Supply Cabinet

A large supply cabinet is an essential piece of training room equipment. This cabinet may be either metal or wood and may be constructed or purchased second-handed. A suitable closet may be used, but it is important that any such storage place be kept locked in order to prevent waste of materials.

Treatment Cabinet

The treatment cabinet must have an adequate working surface and space for holding first-aid supplies for treatment of minor injuries. The cabinet also holds a store of supplies and is kept locked in order to prevent waste of materials and to keep them sanitary. A set of dressing jars placed on the cabinet surface will keep the dressings clean and available. Regular mason jars will suffice. The size of the treatment cabinets varies among schools, but basically a cabinet 78 inches high and 36 inches wide is adequate for most high schools.

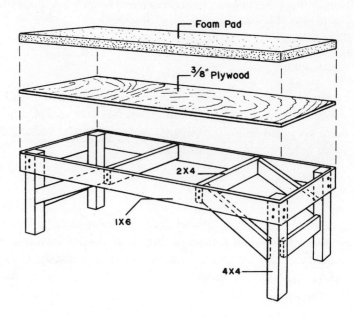

Figure 2-1

Training Table

The training table is the most essential piece of training room equipment. It is used for examining injuries and applying heat, massage, and protective taping or wrapping. Ideally, you need one training table for each 20 athletes. The training table is usually constructed of heavy wood or metal, and its usual measurements are 78 inches long, 24 inches wide, and 30 inches high. The top is covered with foam rubber or some other padding and easily cleaned cloth. A basic training table and its construction pattern is shown in Figure 2-1.

Whirlpool

Another useful piece of equipment for the training room is the whirlpool. It is used for utilizing hot water in motion to care for strains, sprains, and bruises. This piece of equipment should be provided for the training room as soon as possible. However, a hot shower, bucket of hot water, and towels or analgesic packs make good substitutes. One way of improvising a whirlpool bath is to take an old bathtub and use it with a portable water agitator which may be purchased from a local sporting goods dealer or discount house. If the latter is used be certain that the equipment is properly grounded.

A very good method for wet heat application is to use sand filled cloth bags placed in hot water. The sand absorbs and holds heat and provides an inexpensive technique for heat treatments.

SUPPLIES

Training supplies necessary for providing minimal care of the athlete include:

Absorbent Cotton	Antiseptic Liquid
Adhesive Tape	Antiseptic Ointment
Alcohol	Ammonia Capsules
Analgesic Balm	Aspirin Tablets
Antibacterial Soap	Athlete's Foot Solution

Cold Packs
Cold Tablets
Disinfectants
Elastic Wraps
Eye Wash Solution
Felt Rolls and Pads
Foot and Body Powder
Gauze Roller Bandage
Gym Deodorizer
Ichthyol Ointment
Mouthwash

Protective Pads
Rosin Powder
Salicylic Acid
Salt Tablets
Skin Lubricant
Skin Toughener
Sponge Rubber
Swab Sticks
Teeth Protectors
Tongue Depressors

OBJECTIVES

The training table, whirlpool, and other treatment places must be cleaned daily, and floor drains must be kept in operation and cleaned daily.

The athletes should be instructed that the training room is for injury care and that the only persons allowed in the room are those who need this care. The athlete's wear for the training room should be at least a supporter and shower shoes. Fully dressed athletes should not lounge in the room.

SOURCES FOR OBTAINING TRAINING ROOM INFORMATION

In my opinion, your two best sources for obtaining information about building and renovating training rooms can be secured from *The Kendall Company, Bike Sports Division,* 309 West Jackson Boulevard, Chicago, Illinois, and *The Cramer Chemical Company,* Inc., Gardner, Kansas.

3

Skin Injury Care

The most common sports injury is damage to the skin and surrounding tissue. Damages to the skin can be injuries or infections, and in treating these damages, you must keep in mind that maintaining cleanliness, using sterile instruments and materials, and keeping a close watch for infection are basic.

INJURIES

Abrasion

An abrasion is the tearing off of the upper layer or layers of skin; there may be bleeding or oozing of a cloudy substance known as lymph.

An abrasion is caused by scraping the skin against hard objects, such as hard playing surfaces or equipment.

An abrasion may be prevented by keeping the playing area free of all extraneous objects and watering the playing area to keep it soft. The wearing of long-sleeved shirts, long socks, and, for extreme cases, elbow pads or shin guards is often necessary.

An abrasion is treated by washing the wound with soap and water or by having the athlete place the injured area under the shower. After the wound has been thoroughly cleansed, apply an antiseptic healer. For the oozing wound, after thorough cleansing, apply a soothing ointment and sterile dressing.

An abrasion is rehabilitated by daily cleansing of the wound with soap and water and an application of antiseptics or ointments. It is necessary for the wound to remain soft so that it will heal from the inside out. Ointment will prevent the formation of a scab which can be knocked off and thus allow dirt or possible infection to enter the wound.

Blister

A blister is the separation of the outer layer of skin from the inner layer with the intervening space becoming filled with a watery substance or blood.

A blister is caused by friction and pinching, with poorly fitted shoes and socks being the most frequent causes. Dirty socks and poor quality socks and shoes are also suspect.

A blister may be prevented by your seeing that shoes and socks fit properly. You also must see that socks are kept clean and that poor quality shoes are discarded. Application of skin tougheners and the wearing of thin cotton socks under the wool socks will also help. A successful blister prevention method employed by me at the University of Kentucky utilized cold applications, and it completely eliminated blisters. It requires the athlete to report immediately any localized burning sensation and to immerse the affected part in cold water until the burning sensation subsides. The localized burning sensation may also be sprayed with an instant ice solution. Still another preventive measure is application of soothing ointment to be covered with a sterile pad taped to the foot. Moleskin may also be applied to the potential blister area.

A blister is treated by puncturing the wound or removing the skin over the blister. Both methods are accepted procedures, but with either method, extreme care must be taken to use sterile instruments and to maintain cleanliness. After the wound has been drained, the application of an antiseptic and sterile pad with ointment is necessary before resumption of activity. If the athlete has a pair of shower shoes, he wears these when he is not participating so that the blister can get air.

A blister is rehabilitated by keeping the wound clean and covered with antiseptics. While the athlete is engaged in competition, cover the blister with ointment and a sterile pad. Then cut a hole in the felt pad or sponge rubber which is slightly larger than the wound area and tape this to the blister area to prevent friction (Figure 3-1). At other times, apply an antiseptic and keep the wound exposed to the air.

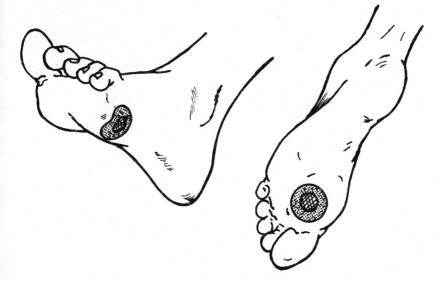

Figure 3-1

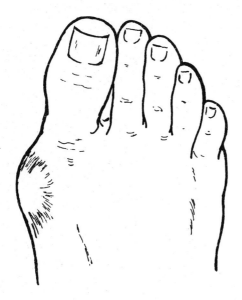

Figure 3-2

Bunion

A bunion is the swelling of the bursae at the jointure of the big toe and foot (Figure 3-2). Its consequences include severe pain, swelling, disability, and possible deformity which is noticeable just inside the ball of the foot when the athlete goes up on his toes.

A bunion is caused by the big toe's being forced inward by shoes that are too short.

A bunion may be prevented by making certain that each athlete's shoes are fitted properly. Ideally, the athlete should purchase his own shoes for assurance of a proper fit. However, when this is not possible many coaches and trainers have the athlete fit his shoes, step in a water filled container, and wear the shoes until they dry. After two or three applications, the shoe will usually conform to the athlete's foot and assure a better fit.

A bunion is treated by restoring the toe to its normal position as quickly as possible without forcing it. Proceed by soaking the toe in warm water or using whirlpool treatments. After drying and cooling the toe, apply skin toughener and a one inch strip of adhesive tape alongside the toe. Gradually pull the tape backward until the athlete notices slight pain; stop at this point and anchor the tape by applying a strip of one and one-half inch tape around the instep (Figure 3-3). Each day apply more pressure until the toe has

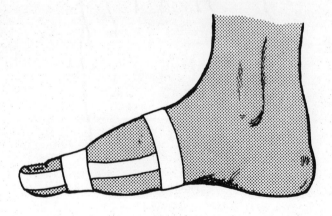

Figure 3-3

returned to normal position. The toe should never be jerked or forced, for if it is, the joint might thus be dislocated. If the athlete already has a deformity, a physician should examine the injury since a bunion often requires corrective surgery.

A bunion is rehabilitated by using the same procedure for treatment with the addition of toe exercises. These exercises consist of the athlete's using his toe to pick a towel or pencil from the floor in order to strengthen the muscles and ligaments and make it easier for the toe to regain normal position.

Burn

A burn is an inflammation of the skin resulting from friction, heat, or acid.

A burn is caused by poorly-fitted pads, dirty supporters, stiff gear, and skin against skin (friction burn); over-exposure to the sun (heat burn); and caustic substances (acid burns).

A friction burn may be prevented by an application of skin lubricant, vaseline, or other lubricant to sensitive areas; a heat burn may be prevented by an application of suntan lotion to exposed areas; and acid burn may be prevented by the use of non-caustic lime or other non-caustic materials.

A burn is treated by applying cold to relieve the burning sensation and then applying a soothing ointment to the burn area. For lime burns, wash the area with soap and water and apply a soothing ointment. In the event of lime burns to the eyes, wash out the eye within 60 to 90 seconds with clear water or an eye wash solution, cover with a sterile gauze pad, and rush the injured athlete to the hospital. Be prepared to treat the athlete for shock* whenever a severe burn occurs.

A burn is rehabilitated by protecting it whenever the athlete is actively engaged in contact or some other form of physical exertion. Be sure that clean, soft clothing is kept near the skin. Eye burn rehabilitation is administered by the physician.

---

* The athlete will experience weakness, faintness, dizziness, and nausea. His breathing may be irregular and shallow; eyes may be vacant and lack-luster with the pupils dilated; pulse may be weak or even absent; and skin may be pale, cold, moist or clammy.

Callus

A callus is a thickened, horny layer of skin which most frequently occurs under the joints of the toes or on the heel of the foot.

A callus is caused by poorly-fitted shoes, poor walking habits, dropped arches, or a protruding bony surface which carries more than its share of weight.

A callus may be prevented by application of skin tougheners, use of metatarsal pads (Figure 3-4), and wearing of properly fitted shoes. The teaching of proper walking techniques and the taping of the arches will relieve tension of the arches and evenly distribute weight. In taping the arches, place a strip of two inch tape under the middle of the arch and gently lift upward and snugly attach it on top of the foot.

A callus is treated by first soaking the foot in a hot water bath and then taking a callus file or piece of sandpaper to remove the loose portion of skin. Apply alcohol to the callus area to keep it sterile. *Never use razor blades to remove the callus.*

A callus is rehabilitated by applying pads to the underside of the foot. The edges of these pads should be tapered so that the bulky

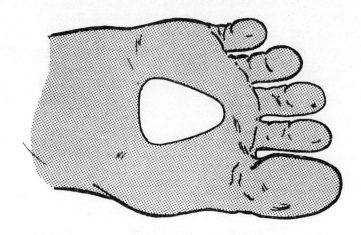

Figure 3-4

part will evenly distribute body weight. Keep the pads in place with the tape.

Chafing

Chafing is an inflammation of the skin resulting from excessive friction. It most frequently occurs between the legs around the groin area.

Chafing is caused by the legs rubbing together, tight pants or supporters, dirty or stiff supporters, excessive sweating, and failure to dry thoroughly.

Chafing may be prevented by applying skin lubricant between the legs and to the groin area, placing cotton in the supporter (Figure ‧3-5), using body powder and proper drying techniques,

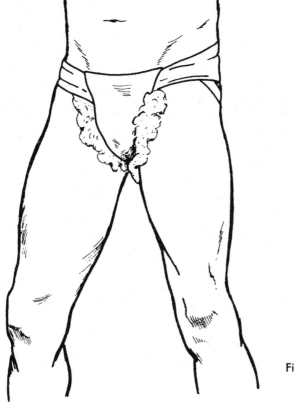

Figure 3-5

wearing clean pants and supporters, and eliminating too tight clothing.

Chafing is treated with alcohol and powder applications. For extreme cases, apply cotton in the shorts to relieve the pressure. Apply antiseptics each day and watch for infection.

Chafing is rehabilitated by applying antiseptics, skin lubricant, and body powder each day before and after practice or competition.

Corn

A corn is a coneshaped, horny layer of skin which usually forms on the upper part of the toe or between the toes.

A corn is caused by pressure from shoes which are too tight in the toe area.

A corn may be prevented by discarding faulty shoes and reducing friction by applying adhesive tape or moleskin over the toe.

A corn is treated by soaking it in hot water for approximately 10 to 15 minutes. Then use a callus file or piece of sandpaper to cut off the softened material. *Never use razor blades to remove the corn.* Cleanliness must be kept in mind as this procedure is followed until the corn is level with the surrounding skin.

A corn is rehabilitated by applying tape, moleskin, or an adhesive bandage over the toe for workouts, and after practice apply salicylic acid on the area. *Watch for signs of infection such as red streaks, tender areas, swelling, and pus.*

Cut

A cut is the forceful breaking of the skin and surrounding tissue which may be superficial or deep. The most common cut occurs over the eye, on the lip, and on the tongue.

A cut is caused by the kick or bump of another player or by the athlete's falling against sharp objects on the playing surface.

A cut may be prevented by protective equipment, proper fundamentals of play, adherence to the rules, and elimination of extraneous objects from the playing area.

A cut is treated by lengthwise washing of the wound with soap and water so that foreign objects will be removed (Figure 3-6), applying an antiseptic, and covering with a sterile gauze pad. Cuts

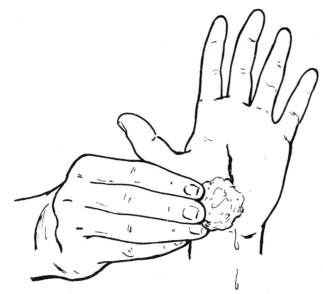

Figure 3-6

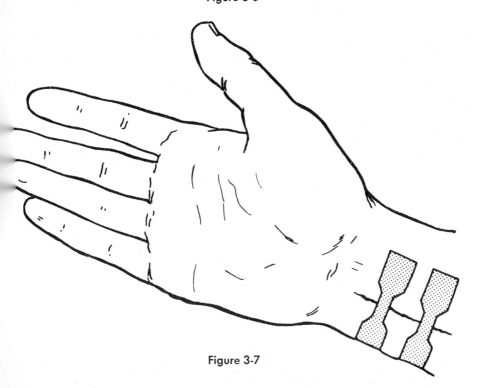

Figure 3-7

on the lip and over the eye often require stitches. In this event, apply a butterfly bandage to close the wound (Figure 3-7), and send the athlete to the physician.

A cut is rehabilitated by using sanitary procedures first of all. Keep the area soft so that a thick scab will not form, and cover the cut with a sterile pad for practice and games. *Keep a close watch for infection.*

SKIN INFECTIONS

Athlete's Foot

Athlete's foot is a frequently occurring infectious disease which affects the feet, especially between the toes. It is usually a chronic, scaly condition with redness and itching between the toes and, in extreme cases, on the bottom of the foot.

Athlete's foot is caused by careless drying habits, the athlete's use of moist, moldy sweat socks, walking barefoot around the shower room, and general lack of cleanliness.

Athlete's foot may be prevented by thorough cleaning of shower and locker rooms, airing and drying of athletic clothing and equipment, and the athlete's regular use of clean socks, athletic supporters, underwear, bath towels, and daily application of foot and body powder.

Athlete's foot treatment requires patience and constant vigilance from both you and the athlete. The use of white cotton socks, changed daily and boiled before using again, is helpful. Other methods of treatment include use of antiseptics, foot ointment, and foot powder. The wisest treatment keeps the socks and feet clean and dry.

Athlete's foot rehabilitative procedures require the use of sanitary techniques, thorough drying of the feet, especially between the toes, and a constant watch to see that the disease does not recur. The athlete must use foot and body powder after each shower and daily put powder in his shoes and socks.

Boil

A boil is a localized staph infection of the skin. It usually starts as an infection around a hair follicle.

A boil results when infections enter through a hair follicle or sweat gland or through a small cut, scratch, or skin abrasion which has not been properly sterilized and treated. A boil may also take root when local resistance is below par.

A boil may be prevented by cleanliness of the body and athletic facilities. If the shower and locker rooms are kept clean, the germs will not have a chance to spread. The use of clean, dry clothing, equipment, and facilities will also help to create a boil-free atmosphere.

A boil is treated by cleaning the boil and all surrounding area within two inches with alcohol or some other antiseptic. Wash the entire area with a sterile gauze pad covered with an antiseptic soap solution. Then prepare a sterile gauze pad with a thick layer of ichthyol ointment and cover the boil area. Apply a skin toughener to the surrounding area and tape the pad in place with cellophane tape. *Never squeeze a boil.* To do so will break down the protective wall and allow the infection to spread throughout the blood stream.

A boil is rehabilitated by repeating the above treatment twice daily until the boil has opened. Then remove the core by placing your fingers at the base of the boil and pressing down and away. Continue daily treatment until the crater has closed and new skin has formed.

Carbuncle

A carbuncle is a group of boils clustered and associated in a local area. Several heads may form at the same time.

A carbuncle, like a boil, is caused by infections of the hair follicles or sweat glands.

A carbuncle's treatment is identical to that for boils; however, the carbuncle requires more thorough care and attention. You must remain aware of the added danger that a carbuncle can cause shock to the nervous system, and therefore, it is advisable for a physician to treat this particular infection.

A carbuncle should be rehabilitated under the physician's supervision.

Cold Sore

A cold sore is an eruption which appears about the mouth and nose.

A cold sore results from common colds or exposures to sunburn or raw, damp cold winds. It frequently follows chapped lips, and it is most often seen in nervous individuals who are continually sucking the lip or bathing the lip with the tongue.

A cold sore may be prevented, in some instances, with the application of Vaseline petroleum jelly, chap-stick or some other lubricant.

A cold sore is treated by first cleaning the area with alcohol and sterile cotton or gauze pad. Then apply a thin coating of skin toughener, powder or some other drying substance. This type of treatment will protect an inflamed area from air and moisture.

A cold sore is rehabilitated by always keeping the area clean and sanitary and following through with one of the suggested treatments. Daily treatment is a must.

Dermatitis

Dermatitis is an inflammation of the skin characterized by intense itching.

Dermatitis is caused by the imprisonment of sweat and skin oils beneath close-fitting clothing or tape. It also results when the athlete is allergic to adhesive tape or skin tougheners or when tape or equipment cause friction.

Dermatitis may be prevented by keeping the skin clean. Supplementary use of skin tougheners, when the athlete is not allergic to it, will prevent dermatitis.

Dermatitis treatment includes removal of adhesive tape with tape remover, washing the infected area with alcohol and mild soap, and application of an antiseptic to the area.

Dermatitis is rehabilitated by requiring extreme cleanliness and follow through of treatment steps.

Dhobie's Itch

Dhobie's itch (jock itch) is an inflammation of the groin area characterized by intense itching. The involved area will often become raw from scratching, which causes severe bleeding and lymph drainage. The danger of infection is great.

Dhobie's itch is caused by careless personal hygiene on the part of the infected individual or of those with whom he associates. The most common cause is the use of a dirty, sweat-stiffened supporter which allows friction and heat to create conditions for the growth of the fungus.

Dhobie's itch may be prevented by the use of extreme care in cleanliness on the part of the athlete. This cleanliness includes a high degree of personal hygiene, prevention of transfer of personal equipment such as supporters, socks, shorts, and shirts, and adequate ventilation of lockers and locker rooms. The use of foot and body powder after thorough drying is helpful in any case. *Care should be taken to keep the powder off the head of the penis.* An extreme case can be prevented by a lubricant to the groin areas and placing of cotton in and around the edges of the supporter. The athlete should wear boxer type shorts under his supporter until the condition has subsided.

Dhobie's itch is treated by thoroughly cleaning the area with soap and water, spraying with germicide and covering with ointment. After the affected area heals, stop ointment treatments and start using daily applications of skin toughener, skin lubricant and body powder.

Dhobie's itch is rehabilitated by requiring constant treatment and adherence to cleanliness. You must be sure that the athletes have clean clothing each day and that infected athletes are applying lubricants and powder before and after activity. The infected athlete should wear cotton in his supporter and boxer type shorts when he is not participating. A close observation should be maintained to prevent serious complications.

Ingrown Toenail

An ingrown toenail is an overlapping of the nail by the adjacent tissue and is often attended by painful ulceration. It is most common in the big toe.

An ingrown toenail is usually caused by the athlete's rounding off the toenail instead of cutting it straight across, and by a downward pressure on the nail and an upward and inward pressure of the flesh. This forcing of the nail to penetrate the flesh is usually caused by improperly fitted shoes or socks.

An ingrown toenail may be prevented by teaching athletes to cut their nails straight across with a slight indentation toward the center of the toe. You should also check to see that the nails are not too short and that the socks and shoes fit.

An ingrown toenail treatment involves soaking the foot in a hot bath to make the toenail more pliable. Then saturate a piece of cotton in an antiseptic and force it under the edge of the nail so that the nail edge will be lifted free from the flesh (Figure 3-8). Antiseptic ointment is applied to the toe and then covered by a thin gauze bandage which should not be bulky. The treatment continues with new cotton being inserted from time to time until the nail has had a chance to grow out of the flesh.

An ingrown toenail is rehabilitated by following the steps for treatment, keeping a close watch for complications and after the nail has grown out of the skin, show the athlete how to cut the toenail. It is advisable to have the athlete come in for periodic checks until there is definitely no chance for complications.

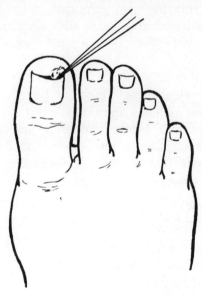

Figure 3-8

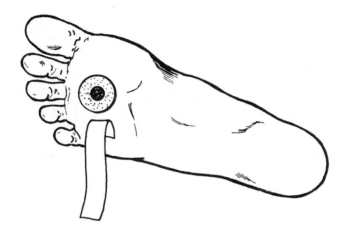

Figure 3-9

Plantar Wart

A plantar wart occurs on the bottom surface of the foot, mostly under the big toe joint or on the heel. The wart differs from a common wart in that it grows inward instead of outward.

A plantar wart's cause is not known, but it is thought that it is caused by irritation from improperly fitted shoes or thin soled shoes which allow bruises to the under surface of the foot.

A plantar wart's first treatment consideration is the elimination of the irritation as completely as possible. Wash the entire foot with soap and water and apply a coating of antiseptic solution, then cut a hole the size of the wart in a piece of felt and apply over the wart area (Figure 3-9). Fill the hole with salicylic acid or an ointment and anchor with adhesive tape over the area. An application of powder on the area will keep it dry.

A plantar wart is rehabilitated by making sure that cleanliness is maintained at all times. Use the steps in treatment for approximately ten days or until the wart has been destroyed. Advise the athlete to check his feet daily and report any recurrence of the plantar wart.

4

Muscle Injury Care

The injury locality most closely associated with the skin is the muscle. However, muscle damages are usually more serious than skin injuries as they may often result in a loss of mobility and sometimes may require surgery. Since muscle injuries will often result in an excessive loss of playing time, it is especially necessary that you become familiar with the methods of preventing, treating, and rehabilitating these injuries.

Whenever a muscle injury occurs, you must take immediate action to reduce swelling and pain with application of cold packs and an elastic wrap. Next day apply heat on the area to increase circulation. The increased circulation will help break up blood clotting formed by excessive bleeding. As soon as pain has subsided, rehabilitative exercises should begin to prevent atrophy (wasting away) of the muscle. Exercises for this purpose include muscle setting, isometric, and isotonic. Muscle setting exercises require the athlete to alternately contract and relax his muscle or muscle groups without causing any body part movement. Isometric exercises require the athlete to hold a muscle or a muscle group in a state of static contraction for a period of six to eight seconds without any body part movement. Isotonic exercises require the athlete to shorten and lengthen his muscles by moving a resistance through a full range of motion. The exercises are repeated daily in order to return the athlete safely back to normal as quickly as possible. Uses of particular rehabilitative exercises will be discussed as applicable to rehabilitation of specific injuries.

Bruise

A bruise is superficial damage to the outer layer of the muscle and is accompanied by pain and discoloration. It is usually mild in nature and will hardly ever keep the athlete from competing.

A bruise is caused by a sharp blow or fall against a hard surface.

A bruise may be prevented with provisions for protective pads needed for contact sports.

A bruise is treated by the application of cold packs. These cold packs are generally left on the bruise area for approximately 15 to 30 minutes in order to stop internal bleeding. Nothing more is done until the next day when heat,* massage, and hot pack are applied.

A bruise is rehabilitated by making sure that the area is properly covered with a hot pack and that there is also protective covering to prevent reinjury. Heat, massage, and hot pack followed by an elastic wrap for support is applied each day until the area is free of pain. The elastic wrap will furnish a slight massage action when the athlete moves from place to place.

Charley Horse

A charley horse results from a bruise of the muscles between the skin and the bone. It is most common on the thigh area (Figure 4-1), and it does not usually show up until the muscle has cooled.

A charley horse is caused by a direct, severe blow to a relaxed or fatigued muscle.

A charley horse may best be prevented by strengthening the muscles, providing salt, and preventing over-fatigue. A fatigued athlete will substitute brief rest periods for alertness, and as he is relaxed during this time he leaves himself open to an unexpected blow.

A charley horse treatment begins while the area is still warm. Stretch the area by having the athlete do a deep knee bend for about one minute. Then apply cold packs for a period of at least 15 to

---

* Generally, heat is applied for 15–30 minutes or until the skin is pink and very warm to the touch.

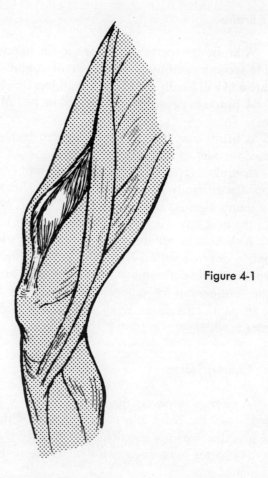

Figure 4-1

30 minutes. After this, wrap the area from the top of the knee to the groin with a charley horse wrap or a wide elastic bandage and advise the athlete to walk around for five to ten minutes. The next day apply heat, massage, and hot packs.

A charley horse is rehabilitated by application of heat and massage for the breaking up of the resultant blood clot. This type of treatment is done once or twice a day, and after each treatment the area is covered with a hot pack. The athlete must frequently stretch the area by doing a deep knee bend in order to prevent stiffening and to relieve the pain of the injured muscle. When the athlete participates, the area must be covered by protective padding. This protective padding is made by cutting a hole in a piece of felt or sponge rubber slightly larger than the charley horse area (Figure 4-2). Place this over the injured area and tape in place. Then cover the entire charley horse area with a football thigh

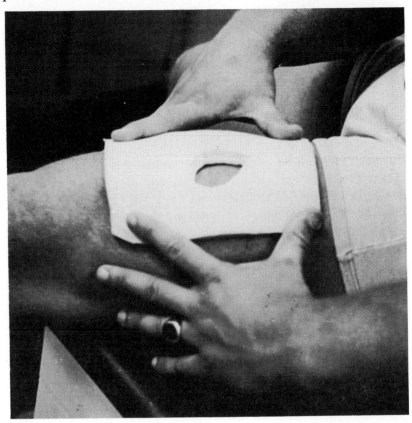

Figure 4-2

pad and wrap the thigh up from the knee to the groin with a charley horse wrap or elastic tape. Closely follow the treatment and rehabilitative process so that calcium deposits will not form.

Muscle setting, isometric, and isotonic exercises are helpful in rehabilitating a charley horse to the quadricep muscles (front thigh). Muscle setting exercises are done while the thigh muscles are so sore movement of the lower leg is impossible. As soon as soreness is reduced, isometric exercises are useful since the muscle can be exercised up to the point of pain and then held for six to eight seconds. The isometric exercise also provides a way to exercise the muscle in different positions without undue harm resulting. When the athlete is able to exert maximum contractions without pain, isotonic exercises provide strength gains from resistance while the body part is moving through a full range of motion.

Muscle setting exercises are done with the athlete assuming a backlying position on the training table. He then alternately contracts and relaxes his thigh muscles for approximately five minutes twice daily.

Isometric exercises are accomplished by having the injured athlete sit on a table so that his lower leg hangs downward at a 90 degree angle to his upper leg. Grasp the front of his ankle and apply sufficient pressure to keep his leg from moving as he tries to extend his knee (Figure 4-3). Next have the athlete straighten his knee to form a 45 degree angle to his upper leg and apply downward pressure as he attempts to straighten his lower leg (Figure 4-4). Then have the athlete straighten his knee. Apply downward pressure as he tries to raise his lower leg (Figure 4-5). Be sure the athlete stretches the exercised area by doing a deep knee bend.

Isotonic exercises are accomplished by having the injured athlete sit on a table so that his lower leg hangs downward at a 90 degree angle to his upper leg. He then moves his lower leg back and forth (extension and flexion) through a full range of motion with a predetermined weight. The athlete chooses a weight that he can successfully lift 10 times. After the first 10 repetitions he rests one and a half times and then does 10 more repetitions, rests one and a half minutes and does 10 more repetitions. The next day he goes through the same routine *with the exception that he rests for only one minute between each set of 10 repetitions.* When the athlete can successfully complete three sets of 10 repetitions with only a minutes rest between sets, he increases his weight load and returns to one and a half minutes rest.

Crick (Wry Neck)

A crick is a spasm of the neck muscles which results in extreme pain when the head is moved. In severe spasm, the neck muscles are fixed and usually swollen resulting in the athlete carrying his head to one side.

A crick is caused by a sudden twist or overflexion of the neck

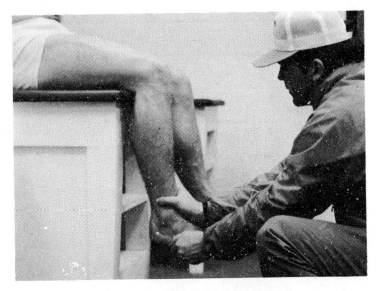

Figure 4-3

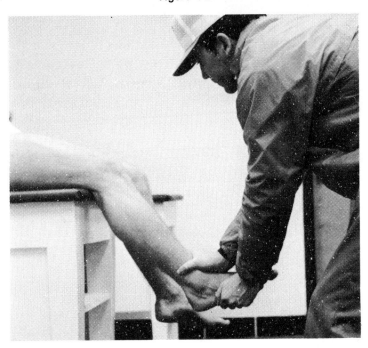

Figure 4-4

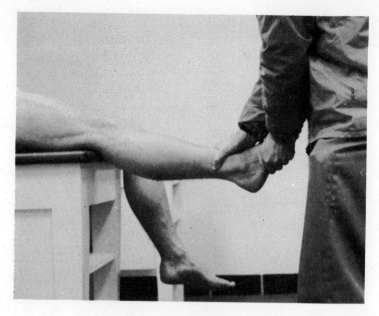

Figure 4-5

or a spinal nerve irritation.

A crick may be prevented by strengthening the neck, upper back, and upper shoulder muscles with the following isometric exercises:

1. Figure 4-6 illustrates the exercise for frontward neck movement. It is administered as follows: Have the athlete lie on his back with arms palms up at his sides. Place one hand on his chest and one hand on his forehead and apply slight downward pressure. Then have him raise his head upward against the pressure in order to strengthen the front and side neck muscles.

2. Figure 4-7 illustrates the exercises for backward neck movement. It is administered as follows: Have the athlete lie on his stomach with arms palms up at his sides. Place one hand on his upper back and one hand on the back of his head and have him raise his head upward against the pressure in order to strengthen the back neck and upper part of the shoulders and back.

3. Figure 4-8 illustrates the exercise for the upper back muscles. It is administered as follows: Have the athlete lie on his stomach and raise his arms upward. Then have him lock his elbows. Apply slight downward pressure at his wrists and have him raise his arms

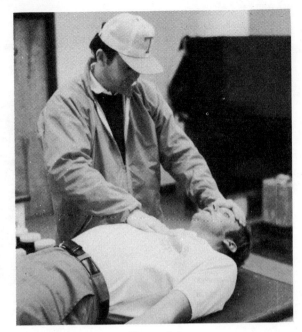

Figure 4-6

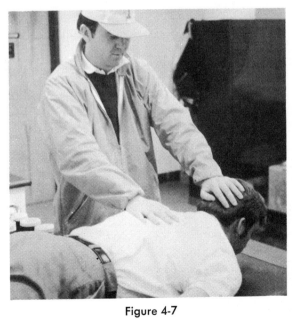

Figure 4-7

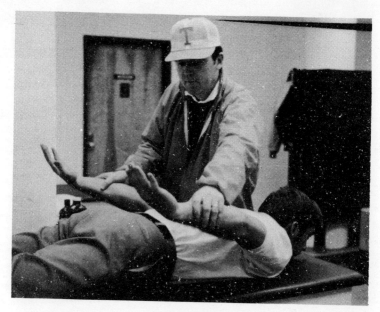

Figure 4-8

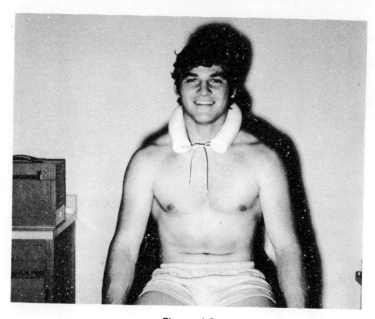

Figure 4-9

against the pressure in order to strengthen the upper back and back shoulder area.

The addition of salt to the diet and the placing of a pad around the athlete's neck will also help in preventing cricks. (Figure 4-9).

A crick is treated by having the athlete lie face down on the training table. Apply heat to relax the muscles and then massage the neck and upper back areas by stretching the muscle tissue away from the spinal column. After completion of the massage, place the athlete on his back with his head near the end of the table. Hold his head in the palm of your hand and gently rotate his head while using your free hand to massage the back of his neck (Figure 4-10). After massaging the neck, isometrically exercise the neck with exercises described on pages 47 and 48. A heat pack for the neck area should be applied to keep it warm.

A crick is rehabilitated by following treatment procedure three to four times each day followed by holding the neck in traction for a period of 15 minutes. Be sure to put the neck in traction only under the careful supervision of the team physician. Usually traction produces immediate relief, but since soreness may last for two to

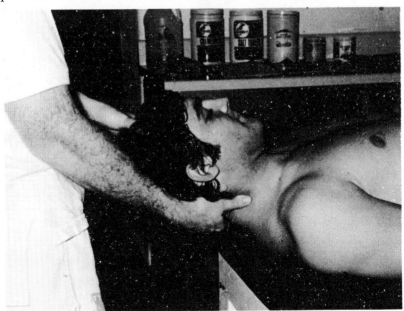

Figure 4-10

three days, it is sometimes necessary to continue rehabilitative techniques for at least three to four days or longer.

Groin Strain

Groin strain is accompanied by pain and will often limit the range of motion of both legs.

Groin strain is caused by the thigh's being spread too far away from the body at the groin.

Groin strain may be prevented by the daily stretching exercise illustrated in Figure 4-11 where the athlete is placing his foot on a table and leaning forward. Increased salt will also help to eliminate groin strain.

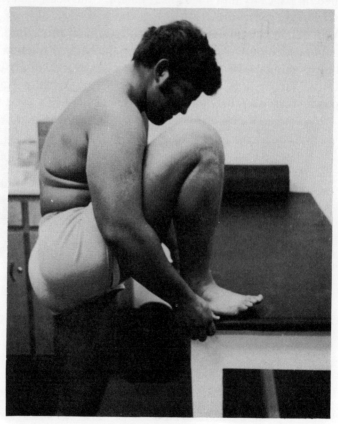

Figure 4-11

Groin strain treatment includes fifteen to thirty minutes of cold packs to the area followed by wrapping an elastic wrap around the leg over the groin area and then around the waist. When the wrap is in place it will resemble a figure-of-eight with the smaller end at the leg and the larger and at the waist (Figure 4-12). The second day's treatment includes heat, massage, and hot pack which is kept on the area until the next day's treatment.

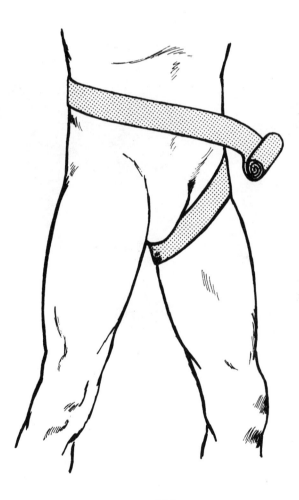

Figure 4-12

Groin strain rehabilitation follows the procedures for treatment. Exercise the area by first having the athlete lie on his back and spread his legs shoulder width apart. Apply pressure to the inside of both ankles and have the athlete resist the pressure by squeezing his legs together (Figure 4-13). Be sure pressure is not exerted past the point of pain. Another good exercise to use has the athlete lying on his back with his feet drawn up to within 12 to 14 inches of his buttocks. Apply inside pressure to the slightly spread knees as the athlete tries to squeeze his knees together (Figure 4-14). These exercises follow the isometric procedure of tension for eight seconds. After exercising, it is important to stretch the groin area by having the athlete place his leg on a table and lean forward (Figure 4-11).

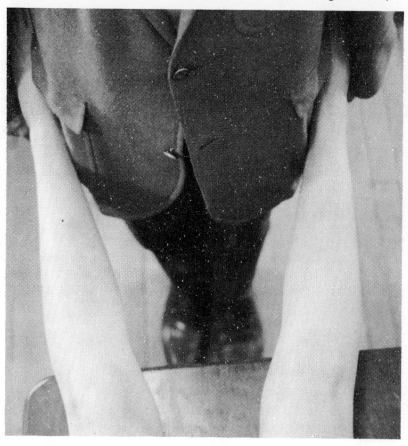

Figure 4-13

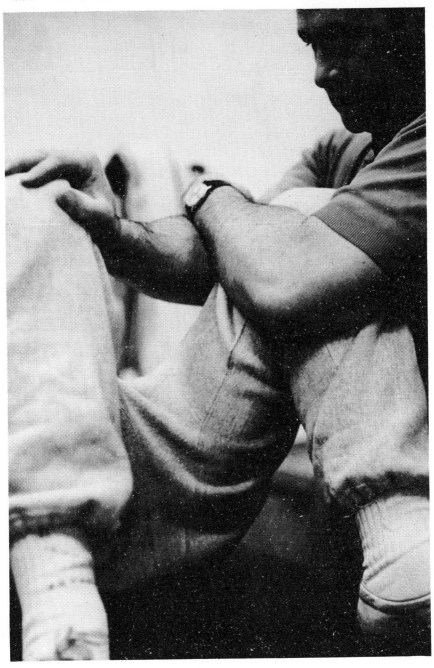

Figure 4-14

Hernia of the Muscle

A hernia of the muscle is an infrequent occurrence in athletics which usually affects the thigh area. It does not interfere with the normal function of the leg and can be controlled with proper bandaging. The hernia appears as a slight bulge when the muscle is relaxed and goes down when the muscle is contracted.

A hernia of the muscle is caused by a severe blow which breaks the covering of the muscle.

A hernia of the muscle may be prevented by wearing of proper protective pads, reduction of over-fatigue, consuming an adequate amount of salt, and strengthening and stretching exercises.

A hernia of the muscle treatment includes the supporting of the injured area with an elastic wrap until the athlete has been seen by a physician who will determine whether surgery is needed. If the physician decides that surgery can wait until the end of the season, protect the area by applying a felt or sponge rubber pad over the area and wrapping with an elastic bandage. For competition, you might cover this bandage with a thigh pad to protect the area from being hit.

A hernia of the muscle rehabilitation begins as soon as the athlete experiences no pain and must be started only with a physician's approval. Isometric exercises are a good method of strengthening the area because they can be stopped at the point of pain and can exercise the muscle at its weakest point.

Spasm (Cramps)

A spasm gives rise to severe pain and short loss of mobility. It is best defined as two muscles pulling against each other.

A spasm is caused by fatigue, cold, upset in salt and water balance through excessive perspiration, a blow, or overstretching of unconditioned muscles.

A spasm may be prevented by prevention of fatigue through well-organized practice and game programs, proper warm-up procedures to prevent cold muscles, strict adherence to the taking of salt, and a good pre-season conditioning program to prevent overstretching of untrained muscles. *Any athlete who is not conditioned should not be allowed to participate.*

A spasm is treated by grasping the muscle firmly with both hands and squeezing as hard as possible until it has subsided. The treatment for spasm differs since it includes as its first treatment *application of heat* to the area and massaging to restore circulation. This will increase the oxygen supply to the area and thereby drain off the pain causing waste products. An application of a hot pack for overnight use is also necessary.

A spasm rehabilitative procedure includes extra salt in the athlete's diet and strengthening and stretching exercises for increased circulation to the affected area. Additionally, the spasm area must be constantly heated and massaged. Whenever there is a large number of muscle spasm experienced by the team, the amount of salt given to each athlete must be increased; this is especially true for hot, humid climates.

Strain

A strain is the tearing of the muscle and is always followed by acute pain and immediate loss of function as well as localized tenderness.

A strain is caused by a violent forcing of the muscles beyond its normal range.

A strain may be prevented by proper conditioning techniques, adequate salt intake, maintenance of smooth playing surfaces and areas, and strengthening and stretching exercises.

A strain is treated by first applying cold packs along with a compression bandage (charley horse wrap, elastic bandage, or elastic tape) for approximately 30 minutes to reduce internal bleeding. After the cold packs have been removed, apply a compression bandage for overnight use. Advise the athlete to put ice on the area whenever possible. He should also elevate the affected part whenever possible. Next day apply heat, massage, and muscle setting exercises. Continue these treatments until the athlete experiences no pain.

A strain is rehabilitated with procedures similar to treatment in that heat, massage, and exercises are carried out. The largest portion of rehabilitation time is devoted to heat and strengthening and stretching exercises. Always keep a hot pack anchored with an elastic wrap on the area until it is completely healed. If the athlete participates, protective pads must be provided.

5

Joint Injury Care

A joint is the junction of two or more bones joined together by the ligaments, lubricated by the bursae, and bound by the tendons. They are open to injury when forced beyond their normal range of motion. This forcing of the joint tends to stretch and weaken the ligaments which when torn or severely stretched will not return to normal without surgery. Therefore, joints that have not been properly treated tend to be loose and more susceptible to disabling injury. Common injuries which affect joints are bursitis, dislocation, fracture, separation, and sprain.

The following suggested procedures will help in the recognization, prevention, treatment, and rehabilitation of joint injuries. Since the joints of the ankle, elbow, hip, jaw, knee, shoulder, and wrist are the most common joint injuries, primary emphasis is given to them.

ANKLE INJURIES

Anatomy

The ankle is a hinge joint formed by the jointure of the lower leg bones with the talus (Figure 5-1). It is stabilized by three powerful ligaments, the inferior tibio-fibular ligament binding the fibula to the tibia, the medial ligament on the inside, and the lateral ligament on the outside (Figure 5-2). Along with these ligaments, there are the tendons of the calf muscles and front leg muscles which form a stirrup for the ankle.

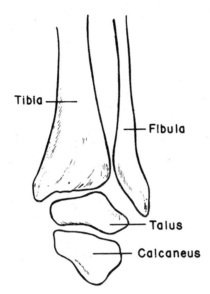

Figure 5-1

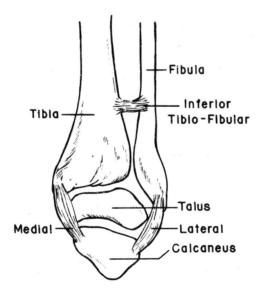

Figure 5-2

Examination

When the ankle is injured, there is a possibility that it may be dislocated, fractured, or sprained. These possibilities must be kept in mind when examining the injury. Look for obvious deformities, for localized tender areas, for limited ankle movement, and for the exact point of injury. Point of injury may be determined with the following manual tests:

1. Figure 5-3 illustrates the downward movement test (plantar flexion) which is administered as follows: With the athlete's foot at a right angle to his leg, firmly grasp his ankle and hold the bottom of his foot. Have the athlete push downward against the pressure in order to test for an injury to the back of the ankle and back leg area.

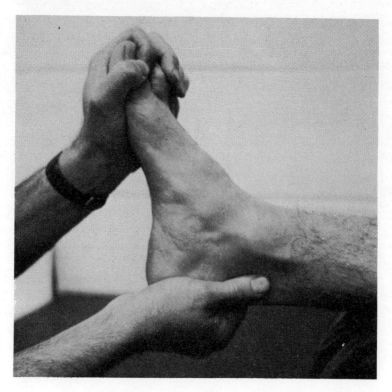

Figure 5-3

2. Figure 5-4 illustrates the upward movement test (dorsiflexion) which is administered as follows: With the athlete's foot in a relaxed position, hold his heel in your palm. With your other hand, hold his foot as he pulls upward against the pressure in order to test for an injury to the area along the front of the leg, ankle, and foot.

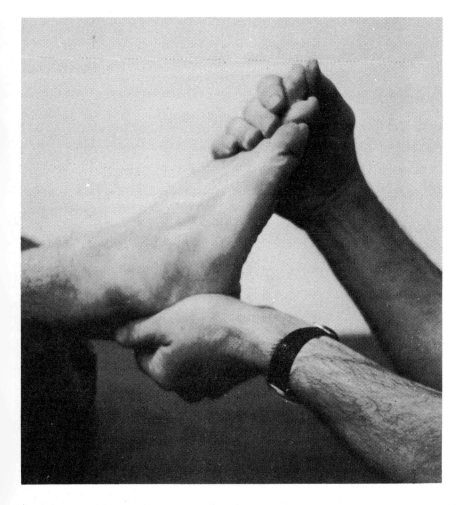

Figure 5-4

3. Figure 5-5 illustrates the inward movement test (inversion) which is administered as follows: With the athlete's foot relaxed, apply pressure to the outside heel area and to the inside toe area. Have the athlete turn his foot inward and pull upward in order to test for an injury to the area along the outside of the ankle and front of the leg.

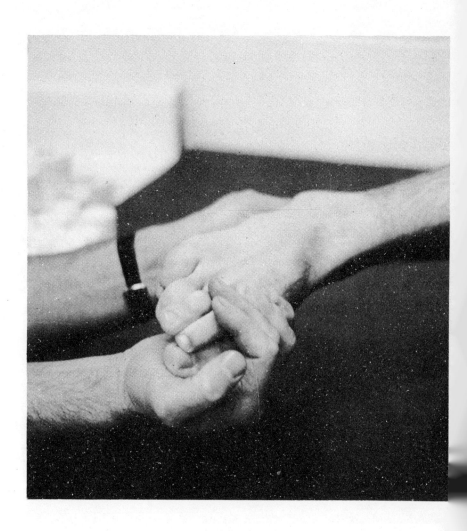

Figure 5-5

4. Figure 5-6 illustrates the outward movement test (eversion) which is administered as follows: With the athlete's foot relaxed, apply pressure to the inside heel area and to the outside toe area. Have the athlete turn his foot outward and pull upward in order to test for an injury to the area along the inside of the ankle and leg.

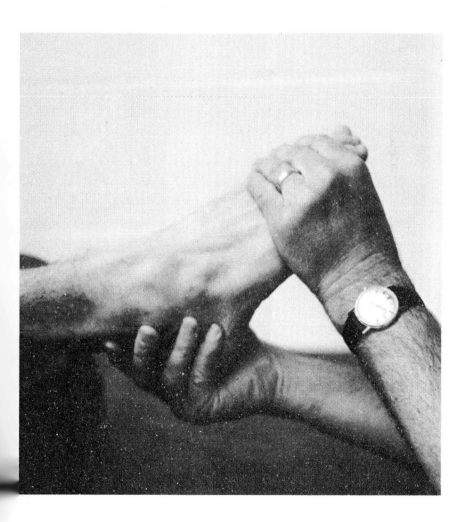

Figure 5-6

Treatment

When no abnormal or undue pain is brought out by the examination and manual tests, tape or wrap the athlete's ankle and allow him to resume practice. Injuries limiting participation for the rest of practice must be promptly and properly treated.

Dislocation   An ankle dislocation is usually obvious and accompanied by pain, loss of movement, and disability. The most common dislocation is backward (Figure 5-7); however, the ankle may also be dislocated forward or sideways.

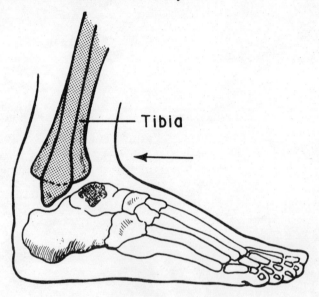

Tibia

Figure 5-7

An ankle dislocation is caused by a severe twisting, over-extension, or binding of the joint as a result of falling, stepping in a hole or being struck by a great force.

An ankle dislocation may be prevented by utilizing exercises to strengthen the muscles which cover the ankle area and to instruct the athletes about the inherent hazards connected with sports. Taping or wrapping the ankle is also considered a good preventive measure.

An ankle dislocation is treated with cold packs, splint, and transportation to the physician. The physician will give further treatment and prescribe rehabilitation procedures.

An ankle dislocation rehabilitation starts when the physician releases the athlete. At this time, the ankle area is heated, massaged, and exercised so that it will again become strong.

Fracture   An ankle fracture is a cracking or breaking of one or more bones which compose the ankle joint. There will be immediate intense pain, localized tenderness, swelling, limitation of movement, muscle spasms, redness, deformity, and harsh grating sensations which may be heard above the joint. The lower ends of the leg bones are the common sites of fracture, and when the fracture is of the small bone (fibula) of the lower leg, it is called Pott's Fracture (Figure 5-8).

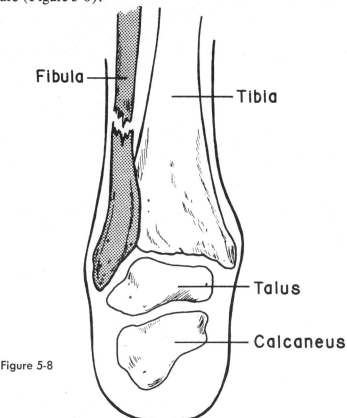

Figure 5-8

An ankle fracture is caused by direct blows, falls, severe twisting or by falling over an extended leg in a pileup.

An ankle fracture may best be prevented by strengthening the muscles around the ankle joint. Use of ankle wraps and tape are considered important preventive measures.

An ankle fracture is first treated by making a true diagnosis of the injury. If it is diagnosed as a fracture, a splint is applied and the athlete transported to a physician for further treatment. When the injury cannot be diagnosed as a fracture, it is treated as a severe sprain and *X-rayed* as soon as possible. The application of cold packs, elastic wrap and elevation of the ankle is also important.

An ankle fracture rehabilitation procedure will be prescribed by the physician.

Sprain   An ankle sprain is the partial or complete tearing of one or more ligaments about the ankle joint. The common classifications of ankle sprains are outward, inward, and forward. The most common is the outward which causes a stretch or rupture of the ligaments on the outside of the ankle. Ankle sprains may vary from slight twists to severe sprains; therefore, the nature of sprains will be different. However, the symptoms of pain, tenderness, swelling, loss of motion, redness, and deformity will usually be the same in all cases.

An ankle sprain is caused by a severe twisting of the ankle joint past its normal range of motion.

An ankle sprain may be prevented by checking of playing surfaces, closer adherence to the rules regarding pile-ups, taping and wrapping the ankle, and pre-seasonal and seasonal strengthening and stretching exercises.

An ankle sprain is immediately treated with an application of cold. This cold may be applied by having the athlete put his foot, shoe and all, in a tub of ice water, use of ice bags, or commercial ice solutions. The ankle is then wrapped with an elastic wrap, covered with an ice pack, and elevated. After the cold pack has been removed, lightly place an elastic wrap on the ankle. Be certain that the wrap is not so tight that it will restrict circulation. In case of a severe sprain, denoted by excessive swelling, deformity, and extensive pain, *X-ray* the joint to check for fracture or dislocation. The next day start heat, massage, hot packs, and exercises.

An ankle sprain rehabilitation includes application of heat, massage, hot packs, and exercise twice daily.

Exercises

Daily exercising of the ankle assures quick return to normal strength. Following is a description of isometric, isotonic, and stretching exercises for this purpose.

Isometric Exercises   Each of the following isometric exercises is done for eight seconds. These exercises follow:

1. The downward action exercise is administered as follows: With the athlete's foot at a right angle to his leg, firmly grasp his ankle and hold the bottom of his foot. Have him push downward against the pressure in order to strengthen the back heel and leg area (Figure 5-3).

2. The upward action exercise is administered as follows: With the athlete's foot in a relaxed position, hold his heel in your palm. With your other hand, hold his foot as the athlete pulls upward against the pressure in order to strengthen the area along the front of the leg, ankle, and foot (Figure 5-4).

3. The inward action exercise is administered as follows: With the athlete's foot relaxed, apply pressure to the outside heel area and to the inside toe area. Have the athlete turn his foot inward and pull upward in order to strengthen the area along the outside of the ankle and front of the leg (Figure 5-5).

4. The outward action exercise is administered as follows: With the athlete's foot at a right angle to his leg, apply pressure to the inside heel area and to the outside toe area. Have the athlete turn his foot outward and upward in order to strengthen the area along the inside of the ankle and leg (Figure 5-6).

5. Figure 5-9 illustrates the straight-legged toe rise which is administered as follows: Have the athlete stand near a table so that he can balance himself. Then have him rise on his toes in order to strengthen the calf muscles (gastrocnemius).

6. Figure 5-10 illustrates the bent-legged toe rise which is administered as follows: Have the athlete stand near a table so that he can balance himself. Then have him bend his knee and rise on his toes in order to strengthen the lower calf muscle (soleus).

Isotonic Exercises   Each of the following isotonic exercises is done as follows: The athlete chooses a weight that he can

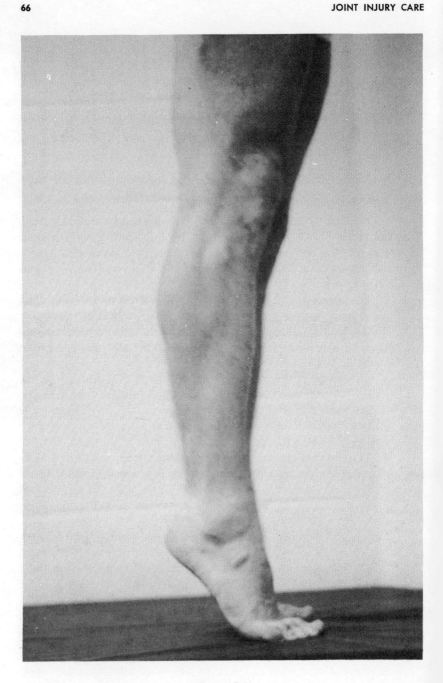

Figure 5-9

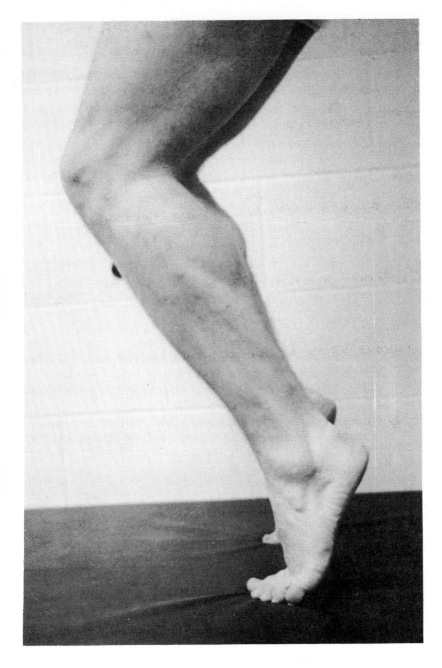

Figure 5-10

successfully lift 10 times. After the first 10 repetitions he rests one and a half minutes and then does 10 more repetitions, rests one and a half minutes and does 10 more repetitions. The next day he goes through the same routine *with the exception that he rests for only one minute between each set of 10 repetitions.* When the athlete can successfully complete three sets of 10 repetitions with only a minutes rest between sets, he increases his weight load and returns to one and a half minutes rest.

The upward and downward movement exercise is administered as follows: The athlete, while seated on a table or lying on his back, moves his ankle up and down through a full range of motion for three sets of 10 repetitions.

The inward and outward turning exercise is administered as follows: The athlete sits on a table so that his lower leg is at a right angle to his upper leg. He then turns his foot inward and outward through a full range of motion for three sets of 10 repetitions.

Stretching Exercises   Each of the following stretching exercises is done 10 times twice a day. These exercises follow:

1. Figure 5-11 illustrates the heel cord stretcher which is administered as follows: Have the athlete stand with his heels flat. Then have him lock his knees and lean forward against a wall while keeping his heels flat on the floor in order to stretch the heel cord and back of the leg.
2. Figure 5-12 illustrates the lateral stretch which is administered as follows: Have the athlete first roll his ankle inward and then outward in order to stretch the inside and outside of his ankle, foot, and leg.

Strapping

After the ankle has been treated and exercised, it must be protected with either a hot pack, wrap, or tape.

Hot Pack   The hot pack's purpose is to provide warmth, increased circulation, and prevention of excessive stiffness to the injured area. *It is never put on an area where the skin is broken.* Make the hot pack by covering the ankle with analgesic balm about the thickness of a penny, cover with a layer of cotton thick enough to hold heat, but not too bulky to hamper getting the shoe on, and secure with an elastic bandage which is snug but not tight enough

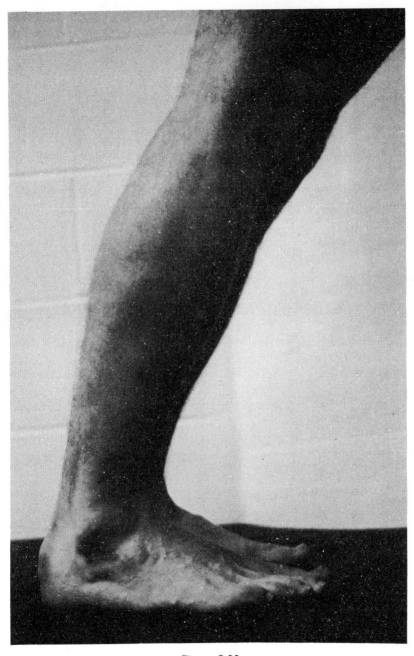

Figure 5-11

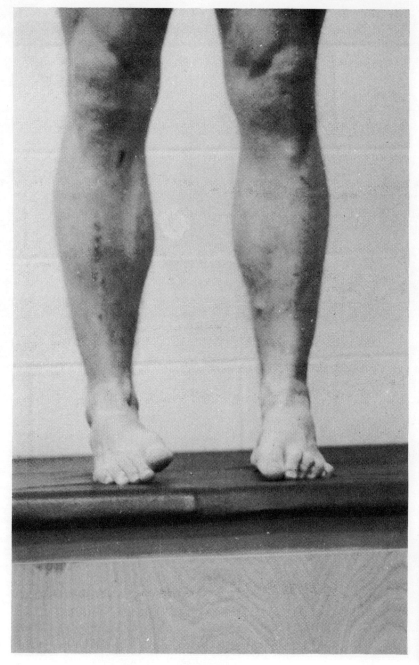

Figure 5-12

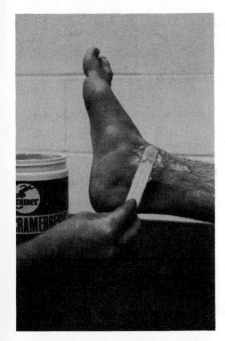

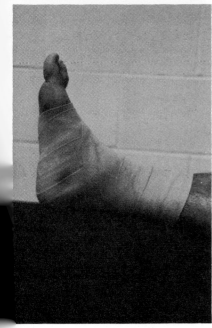

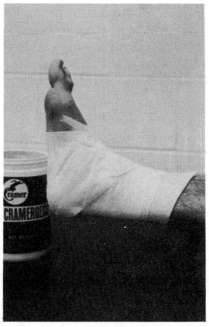

Figure 5-13

to cut off circulation. It is a good practice to continue hot packs for approximately four to five days. Figure 5-13 shows the hot pack application.

Wrapping   The ankle wrap's purpose is to stabilize the ankle joint. It is usually 72 to 96 inches long and can be purchased in bulk form at any sporting goods dealer. For best results, the wrap is put over a sock to prevent friction. Start the wrap high on the instep and move it, at an acute angle to the inside of the foot. From the inside of the foot, move the wrap under the arch coming up on the outside and crossing at the beginning point where it continues around the ankle, hooking the heel. From here, move it up, inside, over the instep and around the ankle, hooking the opposite side of the heel. This completes one series of the ankle wrap. Complete a second series with the remaining material, encircling the ankle. Figure 5-14 shows how the ankle wrap is applied.

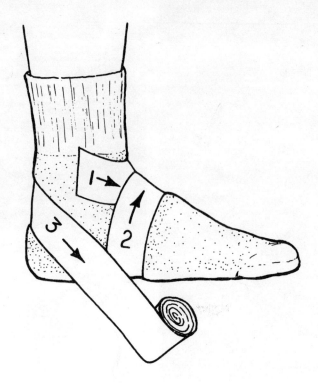

Figure 5-14

Taping Tape is applied to an injured area for protection and promotion of healing. The application of tape requires constant practice and neatness. The beginner should begin slowly and deliberately. Begin preparation for ankle taping by making sure the athlete's ankle is free of hair, clean, and dry. Then have the athlete sit on a table so that his foot forms a right angle to his leg and extends over the edge of the table. Spray the area to be taped with skin toughener, and when the toughener has dried, first apply an anchor strip just below the calf muscle. Then apply a vertical strip from the inside of the leg behind the ankle bone up to the outside of the anchor strip. Next apply a horizontal strip just below the ankle bone. After this is completed apply three more vertical strips and then enclose the entire ankle and leg area with circular strips. Be sure that the tape does not go above the anchor strip. If it does circulation to the leg will be hampered. Also be certain that the tape is *snug but not tight*. Figure 5-15 shows how tape should be applied.

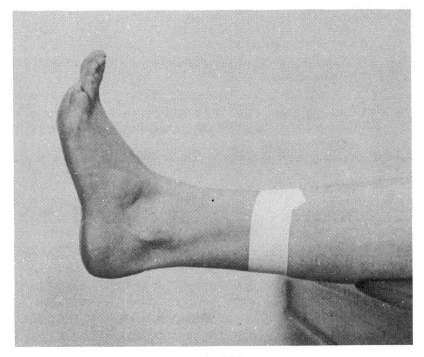

Figure 5-15

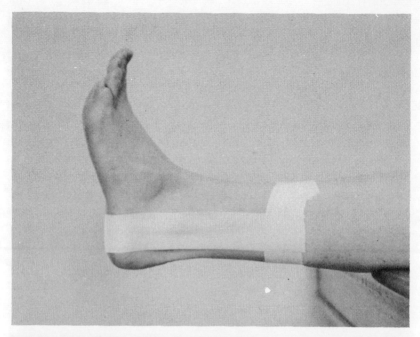

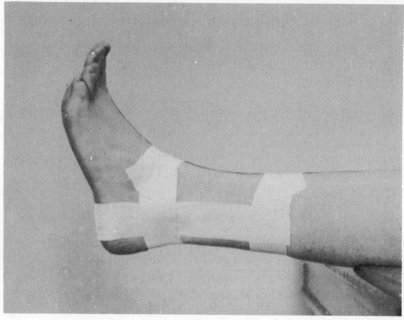

Figure 5-15 continued

ELBOW INJURIES

Anatomy

The elbow is a hinge joint formed by the jointure of the upper arm bone with the lower arm bones (Figure 5-16). It is held in place by the bicep and tricep muscles and by strong ligaments (Figure 5-17) which bind together the two lower arm bones.

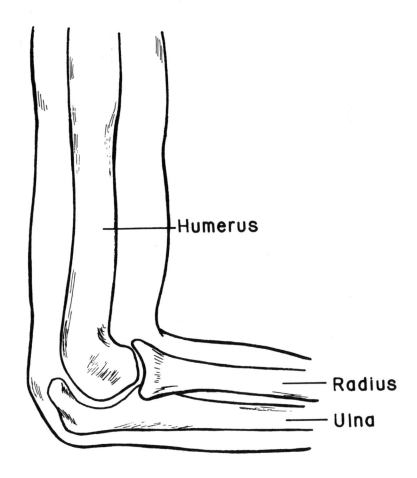

Figure 5-16

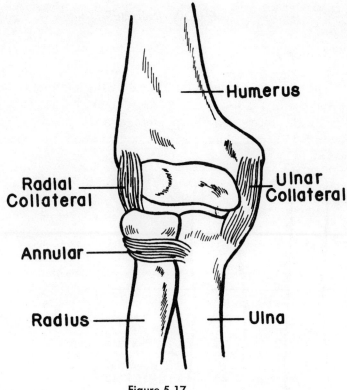

Figure 5-17

Examination

An elbow injury, when improperly handled, can cause a great deal of lost time. Therefore, it is important for elbow injuries to be properly diagnosed by checking for tender areas, deformities, and point of injury. Point of injury may be determined with the following manual tests.

1. Figure 5-18 illustrates the test for the biceps muscle. It is administered as follows: Have the athlete bend his lower arm so that it forms a right angle with his upper arm. Then have him turn his palm up. Grasp his hand and try to pull his arm away from his body as he furnishes an upward pull.

2. Figure 5-19 illustrates the test for the triceps muscle. It is administered as follows: Have the athlete bend his arm so that it

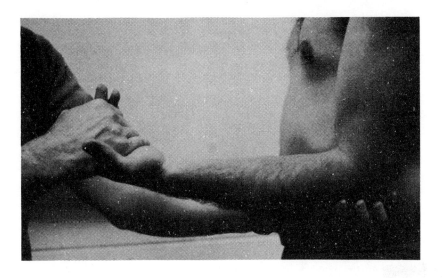

Figure 5-18

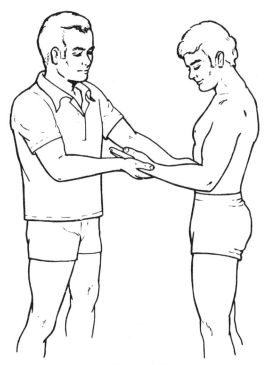

Figure 5-19

forms a right angle with his upper arm. Then have him turn his palm up. Place your hand under the back of his hand and with your other hand stabilize his elbow. Then while the athlete tries to straighten his arm apply slight pressure.

3. Figure 5-20 illustrates the test for the forearm muscles. It is administered as follows: Have the athlete grasp your hand as if he were shaking it. Then have him first try to turn his palm in and then out.

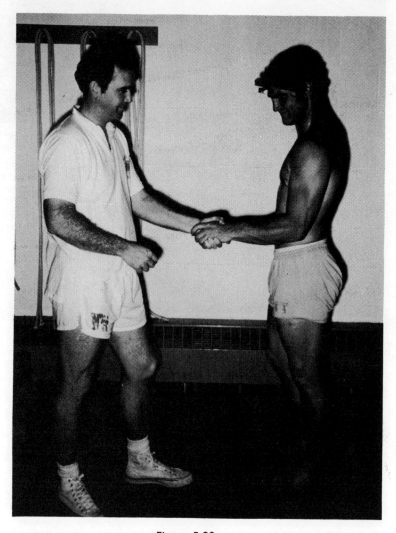

Figure 5-20

Treatment

Elbow injuries commonly connected with athletics are bursitis, contusion, dislocation, epicondylitis humeri (pitcher's elbow, tennis elbow, or golfer's elbow), fracture, hyperextension, and sprain.

Bursitis   Elbow bursitis is an inflammation of the bursa sac. There will be pain, swelling, and limitation of movement. Bursitis will manifest itself as a localized mass under the elbow joint. It may feel hot to the touch and seem extremely tight when pressure is applied.

Elbow bursitis is generally caused by a fall or a sharp blow to the elbow.

Elbow bursitis may be prevented by wearing pads when the athlete plays on hard ground and the watering of the playing area to keep it soft.

The elbow bursa is a self-limiting sac and its secretion will stop when the sac is filled; consequently, there is not much that can be done immediately. The best treatment is to apply cold packs and an elastic wrap for a period of 12 to 24 hours. At the end of this time, heat, massage, exercise (if not too painful), and hot packs are administered. Ultrasound or diathermy is effective, but constant treatment is a must. Some physicians will draw out (aspirate) the excess fluid, but if the bursitis continues, it will probably require surgery for correction.

Elbow bursitis rehabilitation includes the use of heat, massage, hot packs, and exercise. The athlete should be fitted with a sponge pad when he participates. Figure 5-21 shows a way of protecting the bursa area.

Contusion   An elbow contusion is a bruise involving the tissue around the joint. There will be immediate, intense pain and swelling. Shortly, the intense pain will turn to a dull ache that disappears when the elbow joint is at rest.

An elbow contusion is caused by a sharp blow to the elbow when the athlete is hit or falls.

An elbow contusion is best prevented with an application of padding to the elbow area.

An elbow contusion is treated with an application of cold

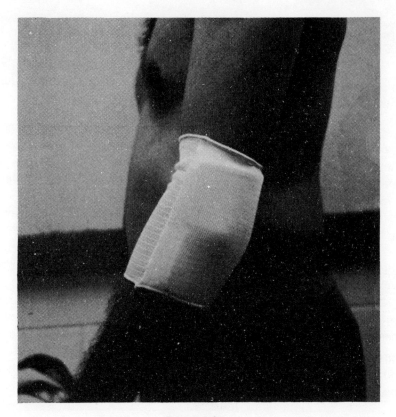

Figure 5-21

packs, pressure with an elastic wrap over a sponge, and a sling so that the elbow can have complete rest. Next day apply heat, massage and elastic wrap over a hot pack.

Dislocation   An elbow dislocation involves one or both the bones of the forearm. The most common dislocation is the backward dislocation that results in the lower arm bones being pushed back of the upper arm bone (Figure 5-22). An obvious deformity will be present above the joint. There will also be loss of function and immediate swelling.

An elbow dislocation is caused by a fall while the arm is straight, a severe counter joint motion (bending backward) or a twist of the arm that involves an unusual motion of the joint.

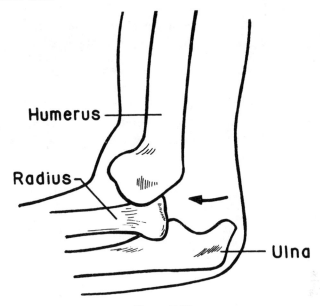

Figure 5-22

An elbow dislocation may be prevented through the teaching of correct falling techniques, fundamentals of play, and exercises for building strength.

An elbow dislocation is treated with an application of cold, splints, and an elastic wrap. Then place the injured elbow in a sling and transport the athlete to the doctor. When the doctor releases the athlete, heat, massage, hot packs, and mild exercises are started. Care should be taken so as not to re-injure the dislocated area.

Epicondylitis   Elbow epicondylitis affects the lower ends of the large bone of the upper arm (humerus). When the pain affects the inside portion of the upper arm bone, it is called "golfer's elbow." Pain on the outside portion of the upper arm bone is often called "pitcher's elbow," "fencer's elbow," or "tennis elbow." Regardless of the exact location of the injury the symptoms are the same. There will be intense pain, tenderness and loss of movement because of weakness. Twisting of the forearm will increase the pain.

Elbow epicondylitis may be prevented by limitation of activity when the elbow becomes overly-fatigued.

Elbow epicondylitis is treated as follows: If it is seen early enough, immediately apply cold packs and a sling. If it is a day old, apply a sling and send the athlete to a physician.

Fracture   An elbow fracture may involve the bones of the upper arm or the bones of the lower arm. A deformity occurs but it is not always visible. In such cases feel the arm for tenderness around the joint and to determine whether or not it is deformed.

An elbow fracture is caused by a sharp, twisting blow from a fall or blow.

An elbow fracture is immediately treated by an application of a splint and a cold pack. The injured arm is then placed in a sling, and the athlete is transported to a physician.

Hyperextension Sprain   A hyperextension sprain is the stretching or tearing of soft tissue around the front of the elbow. There may or may not be swelling, but there will be sharp pain and loss of motion.

A hyperextension sprain is caused by the elbow's being forced beyond its normal range of motion when the arm is straight. The injury occurs in a fall, arm tackling in football, or being caught between two athletes in basketball.

A hyperextension sprain may be prevented by strengthening and stretching exercises and execution of proper fundamentals of the involved sport.

A hyperextension sprain is treated with cold, compression, and a sling. Next day apply heat and have the athlete move his lower arm through a full range of motion. If he cannot fully straighten his arm, apply more heat and manually try to straighten his arm by placing one hand on his elbow and one in his hand and applying pressure. However, be certain that you do not place too much pressure and re-injure his elbow.

A hyperextension sprain is rehabilitated by following treatment procedures for approximately five to seven days at which time isometric exercises can be started. Provide a tape checkrein when the athlete participates.

Sprain   An elbow sprain is similar to the hyperextension sprain in that it is a stretching and tearing of the soft tissue around the joint. It differs from hyperextension sprain since there may be swelling in front, in back, or all around the joint. There will be severe pain when the athlete turns his palm up or down. The athlete will, when in motion, carry his arm by grasping his wrist with his other hand and will be very reluctant to let go.

An elbow sprain is caused by a sudden wrench of the elbow while it is in full extension or full flexion. These conditions might occur when the athlete falls, is caught between two athletes, arm tackles, or is caught by the arm resulting in a twist.

An elbow sprain may be prevented by strengthening and stretching exercises and teaching of proper falling and tackling techniques.

An elbow sprain is treated with cold, compression, and a sling. It should be X-rayed when there is deformity around the joint. Next day apply heat, range of motion movements, and hot packs.

An elbow sprain is rehabilitated by application of heat, range of motion movements, exercises, and hot packs. During this rehabilitation period, be sure that you do not try to make the athlete use the elbow too quickly for if you do it will result in further injury.

Exercises

Following is a description of isometric and isotonic exercises for rehabilitating the elbow.

Isometric Exercises   Each of the following exercises is done for eight seconds twice daily.

The exercise for the biceps muscle is administered as follows: Have the athlete bend his elbow so that his lower arm palm up forms a right angle with his upper arm. Place one hand in his palm and with your other hand stabilize his elbow. Then apply pressure as he tries to bend his elbow (Figure 5-18).

The exercise for the triceps muscle is administered as follows: Have the athlete bend his elbow so that his lower arm palm up forms a right angle with his upper arm. Place one hand under the back of his hand and with your other hand stabilize his elbow. Then apply pressure as he tries to straighten his arm (Figure 5-19).

The exercise for the forearm muscle is administered as follows: Have the athlete bend his elbow so that his lower arm thumb up forms a right angle with his upper arm. Then grasp his hand as if you were shaking it and apply pressure as he tries to turn his palm down and as he tries to turn his palm up (Figure 5-20).

Isotonic Exercises   Each of the following exercises is done according to the directions described on page 65.

Figure 5-23 illustrates the exercise for the biceps muscle. It is administered as follows: Have the athlete sit on a table and grasp a weight so his palm is up. Then have him bend and straighten his arm without changing the position of his palm.

Figure 5-24 illustrates the exercise for the triceps muscle. It is administered as follows: Have the athlete lie face down on a table so that his elbow is at the edge of the table. He then grasps a weight so that his palm is toward his feet and straightens his elbow to full extension and returns the weight to its original starting position.

Figure 5-25 illustrates the exercise for the forearm muscle. It is administered as follows: Have the athlete sit at a table so that the lower arm forms a right angle with his upper arm and is supported by the table. His wrist should extend approximately 12 inches over the edge. Then with his palm up have him grasp a weight and first turn his palm down and then up.

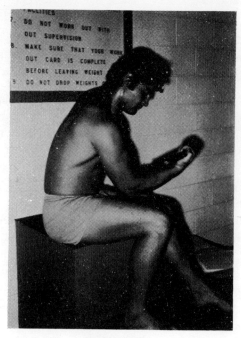

Figure 5-23

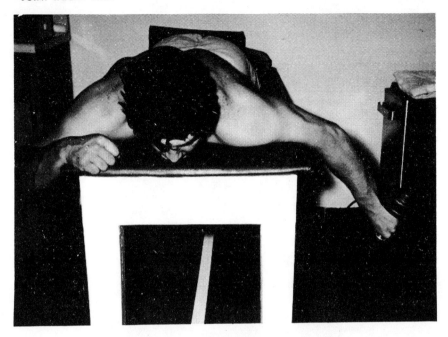

Figure 5-24

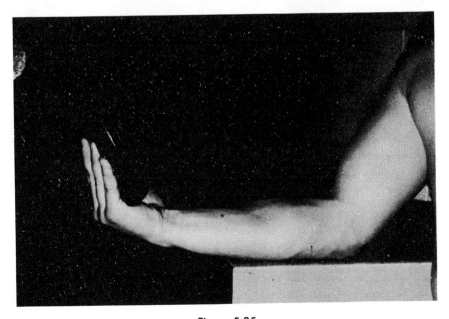

Figure 5-25

Strapping

Hot Pack   Make the elbow hot pack by putting analgesic balm all around the elbow, covering with a layer of cotton, and wrapping with an elastic wrap. Figure 5-26 illustrates an elbow hot pack application.

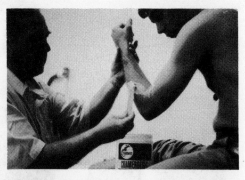
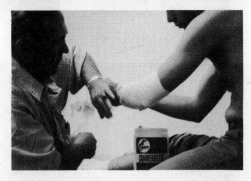
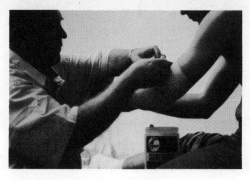

Figure 5-26

Taping   Prepare the area to be taped by shaving off the hair approximately six inches above and below the center of the joint. Then follow the appropriate technique given below.

The hyperextension sprain requires a particular taping technique different from that needed to stabilize the regular elbow sprain. The hyperextension sprain elbow taping, illustrated in Figure 5-27, is applied as follows: Have the athlete slightly bend

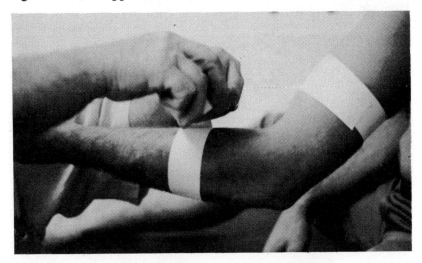

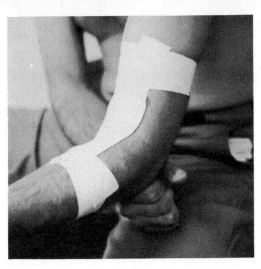

Figure 5-27

his elbow. Place one circular anchor strip above and one below the joint. Next apply about six vertical strips from the top anchor strip across the middle of the joint to the bottom anchor strip. Place circular strips from the bottom anchor strip just short of the bottom of the joint, skip over the joint, and continue circular strips up to the top anchor strip. Make sure the athlete cannot fully straighten his arm. Then cover the entire taped elbow area with an elastic bandage.

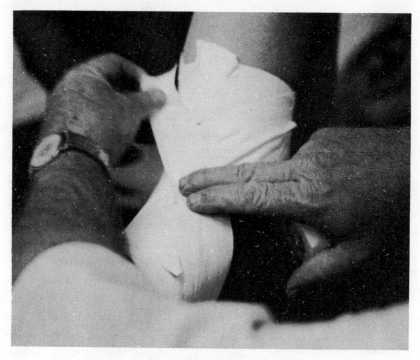

Figure 5-28

Elbow injuries other than hyperextension sprains are taped as follows: Have the athlete bend his elbow slightly. Place one anchor strip below the joint and one above the joint. Next place vertical strips from the top anchor strip to the bottom anchor strip so that they form an "x" over the front center, inside center, and outside center of the joint. Then fully encase the elbow *except the back point* with circular strips of tape and an elastic bandage. Figures 5-27 and 5-28 illustrate the taping technique for elbow sprains.

HIP INJURIES

Anatomy

The hip is a ball-and-socket joint formed by the jointure of
the head of the upper leg bone (femur) with the hip bone socket.
It is held together by strong ligaments and muscles which stabilize
it in four directions making it strong, well-protected, and very
moveable.

Examination

Whenever the athlete complains of pain in the hip area, you
must quickly learn where he is hurting as well as how he was hurt
while making a visual examination of the hip area. Look for
obvious deformities, for localized tender areas, and for limited
movement. Should you note a deformity, immediately immobilize
the athlete by applying a splint and transport him to a physician.
Always watch for signs of shock since it is quite common in hip
injuries.

Treatment

When your examination reveals no serious deformities, check
for one of the following injuries.

Bursitis   Hip bursitis affects the protrusion of the upper
leg bone just below where it joins with the hip bone socket; it also
hinders the tendons and muscles in this area. It will be very painful
and will limit movement. In extreme cases there will be complete
loss of movement. Generally, you will be able to detect heat when
feeling the area just below the hip joint.

Hip bursitis is caused by a severe blow to the area just below
the hip joint when the athlete falls or is hit.

Hip bursitis may be prevented by wearing protective padding
when involved in sports conducive to falls or blows.

Hip bursitis is immediately treated by applying cold packs to the area for two or three days along with rest. The length of cold and rest treatments is dictated by the severity of the injury. After the hip joint cools, start heat treatments and light exercise. Be sure that you do not make the athlete work when there is a sharp pain upon movement.

Hip bursitis is rehabilitated with application of heat, massage, and exercises. Always make certain you do not over-extend the athlete during the rehabilitative stage.

Contusion   A hip contusion is a bruise involving the tissue, muscle, tendons, or bone around the outside hip area. There is pain on movement, and disability varies from one day to ten days.

A hip contusion is caused by blows to the hip area when the athlete hits the playing surface.

Hip contusions may be prevented by wearing protective padding and by keeping playing areas clear of all obstructions that might cause falls.

A hip contusion is treated with immediate application of cold to reduce internal bleeding. Next day apply heat, massage, and light exercises. You must always be aware that hip contusion might develop into bursitis. Usually hip contusion will not cause the athlete to be disabled for more than a few hours.

A hip contusion is rehabilitated by repeated heat treatments and light exercises. Be sure the area is protected for activity by taking a piece of sponge rubber, cutting a hole slightly larger than the tender area, placing it over the injured area, and wrapping with an elastic wrap.

Dislocation   A hip dislocation is a displacement of the upper leg bone from the hip bone socket. There will be an obvious deformity either in the front or back of the hip. The athlete will be immediately disabled and will resist any attempts to move his leg since it causes severe pain. His leg will be turned inward so that his knee and foot tends to rest on his other leg (Figure 5-29).

A hip dislocation, although very rare in athletes, is caused by a severe twisting of the leg.

Hip dislocation may be prevented by strengthening and stretching exercises, by observing rules of play, and by keeping playing areas free of holes and extraneous objects which could

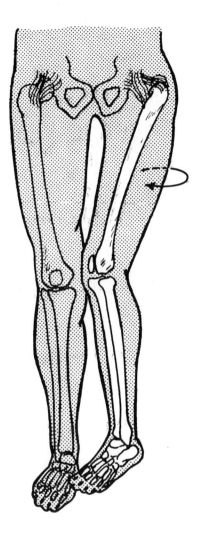

Figure 5-29

cause the athlete to place a severe twist on the hip joint.

Hip dislocation is treated by immediate immobilization of the athlete, application of a splint (Figure 5-30) and transportation to the hospital. You must never attempt to reduce the dislocation since there may be a fracture of the upper leg bone.

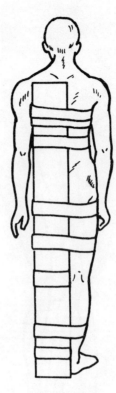

Figure 5-30

Hip dislocation rehabilitation is supervised by the physician. When he gives the word, you begin exercises.

Fracture   A hip fracture is not very common in athletes, but when it does occur, it generally affects the top part of the upper leg bone where it joins the hip bone. There will be severe pain on movement, and in most cases there will be loss of movement.

A hip fracture is caused by twisting the hip joint as in dislocation or by a fall which drives the head of the upper leg bone into the hip socket.

Hip fracture may be prevented by strengthening the hip muscles and by adherence to rules. In sports, especially gymnastics, where there might be a chance of injury to the hip, you should have spotters and you should place protective mats around the playing area.

Hip fracture treatment begins by applying a splint and transporting the athlete to the physician who will make the final evaluation of the extent of injury. You should ask for X rays of any hip injury which results in loss of movement.

Pointer   A hip pointer is a bruise to the top of the hip bone. It causes pain on movement or when the athlete coughs or laughs. It might in very extreme cases cause loss of movement.

A hip pointer is caused by a blow to the top of the hip bone when the athlete falls or is hit by another athlete or by a thrown object.

A hip pointer may be prevented by wearing protective padding.

A hip pointer is first treated with cold packs and an elastic wrap. Next day apply heat massage, and hot packs. Constantly keep the area covered with a hot pack.

Hip pointer rehabilitation follows treatment procedures of heat, massage, and hot packs. For practice or games, protect the area by cutting a hole in a piece of sponge rubber slightly larger than the hip pointer and anchoring with an elastic wrap. Light exercises are also begun at this time.

Sprain   A hip sprain is the stretching or tearing of soft tissue, ligaments, or muscles around the hip joint. There will be localized tenderness and some loss of movement.

A hip sprain is caused by a severe twisting of the hip joint while the leg is planted on the ground. Slipping on a wet floor or field may also cause a hip sprain.

Hip sprain may be prevented by strengthening the muscles that stabilize the hip joint, wearing shoes which prevent slipping or sticking, and keeping playing areas dry and free of extraneous objects.

A hip sprain is treated with immediate application of cold and compression bandage. If the sprain is severe (determined by the team physician), have the athlete rest. For sprains not requiring bed rest, next day apply heat, massage, and passive exercise.

Hip sprain rehabilitation includes the use of heat, massage, and exercise. Rehabilitation of the hip sprain will go very smoothly and quickly if you do not force the rehabilitative stage.

Exercises

Following is a description of isometric and isotonic exercises for rehabilitating the hip joint injury.

Isometric Exercises   Each of the following isometric exercises are done for eight seconds twice daily.

Figure 5-31 illustrates the exercise for strengthening the muscles which move the leg outward (abduction) at the hip joint. It is administered as follows: Have the athlete lie on his back with his arms palms up at his sides. Stand in front of him so that he can rest his ankles on your hips. Then grasp the outside of his ankles and have him try to move his legs outward.

The exercise for strengthening the muscles which move the leg inward (adduction) at the hip is administered as follows: Have the athlete assume the same position described in Figure 5-31. Then have him squeeze inward against your hips.

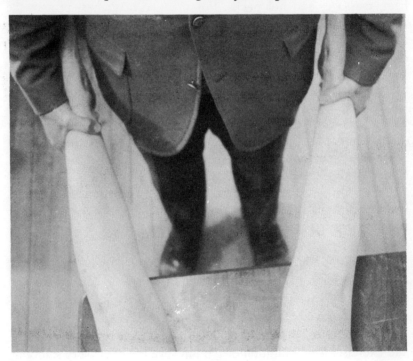

Figure 5-31

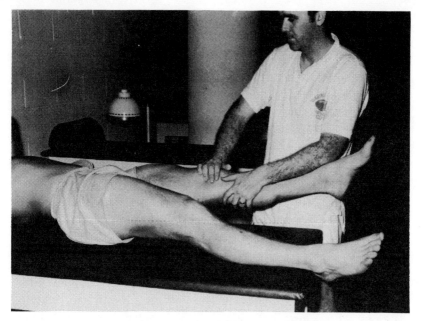

Figure 5-32

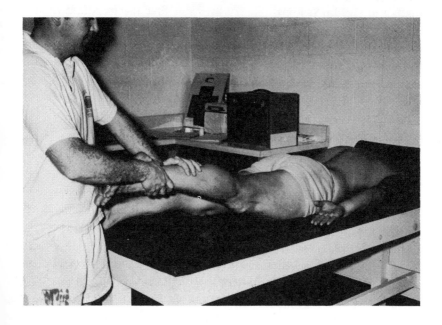

Figure 5-33

Figure 5-32 illustrates the exercise for strengthening the muscles which move the hip toward the front of the body (flexion). It is administered as follows: Have the athlete lie on his back with his arms palms up at his sides. Stand in front of him, grasp his thigh at the knee joint, and apply pressure as he tries to raise his legs upward toward his head.

Figure 5-33 illustrates the exercises for strengthening the muscles which move the hip toward the back of the body (extension). It is administered as follows: Have the athlete lie face down with his arms palms up at his sides. Stand behind him and place your hand on his lower leg. Apply pressure as he tries to raise his thighs upward toward his back.

Figure 5-34 illustrates the exercise for strengthening the muscles which rotate the leg at the hip joint. It is administered as follows: Have the athlete lie on his back with his arms palms up at his sides. Have him turn his foot inward as far as possible. Grasp his foot and his leg at the knee joint and have him try to rotate his leg outward against your pressure. Next have him turn his foot straight up so it forms a right angle with his leg. Grasp his foot and his leg at the knee joint. Then have him first try to rotate his leg inward and then outward. Finally have him turn his foot outward as far as possible. Then grasp it as described above and have him rotate his leg inward.

Isotonic Exercises   Each of the following exercises are done according to the directions described on page 65.

Figure 5-35 illustrates the exercise for strengthening the muscles which move the leg at the hip outward (abduction) and inward (adduction). It is administered as follows: Have the athlete stand close to a table so he can maintain his balance. With a weight attached to his foot, he should keep his knee straight as he first moves his leg at the hip outward and then inward.

Figure 5-36 illustrates the exercise for strengthening the muscle which moves the hip upward toward the front of the body. It is administered as follows: Have the athlete stand close to a table so he can balance himself. With the weight attached to his foot, he should bend his knee so that his upper leg forms a right angle with his body. Then have him raise his upper leg to his body and then lower to the starting position.

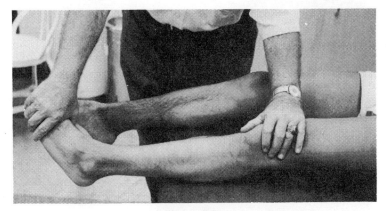

Figure 5-34

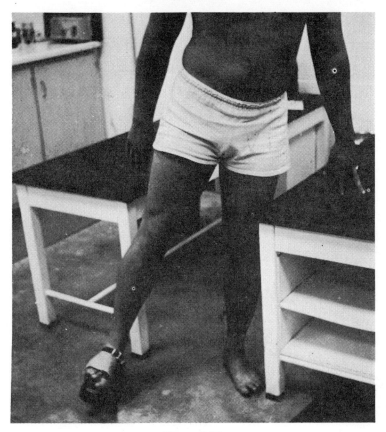

Figure 5-35

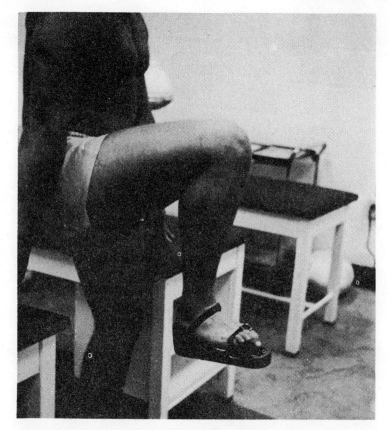

Figure 5-36

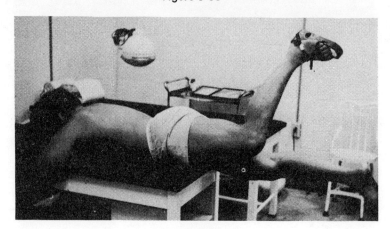

Figure 5-37

Figures 5-37 illustrates the exercise for strengthening the muscle which moves the hip upward toward the back of the body. It is administered as follows: Have the athlete lie face down on a table so that his hips are resting on the end of the table and he is grasping the edges of the table. With a weight attached to his foot, he should bend his knee so that his upper leg forms a right angle with his body. Then have him raise his leg upward toward his body as far as possible and return his leg to its starting position.

Strapping

Hot Pack   Make the hip hot packs by putting analgesic balm on the injured hip area, covering with a layer of cotton, and wrapping with an elastic wrap.

Wrapping   The hip injury is wrapped with an elastic wrap as follows: Start the wrap above the hip joint about even with the lower abdomen. Bring the wrap down at an angle behind the leg, around the buttocks, and around the waist. Then continue down around the leg and back around the waist until the wrap has been completely unwound. Figure 5-38 illustrates the completed wrap

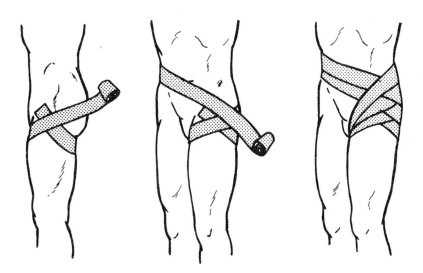

Figure 5-38

which is used for all hip hot packs and compression bandages. Practice is necessary to achieve the correct angles.

Taping   Prepare the area to be taped by shaving off the hair, cleaning with alcohol or antiseptic soap, and spraying with skin toughener. You should use elastic tape for all injuries to the hip joint. Figure 5-39 illustrates the taping technique for the hip pointer. It is applied as follows: Spray the area to be taped with skin toughener. Then place four or five vertical strips of tape from just above the top of the hip to just below the hip joint. Next apply strips of tape at an angle from the bottom of the buttocks to the front of the body just below the ribs and from lower front to upper back so they form an "X" over the top of the hip. Then cover this area from the top of the hip to the area just below the hip with horizontal strips.

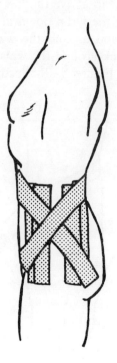

Figure 5-39

JAW INJURIES

Anatomy

The jaw is formed by the jointure of the jaw bone with the base of the skull. It is a supple hinge joint held together with ligaments and muscles, which is vulnerable to blows.

Examination

When the athlete is hit about the face and complains of pain in the jaw area, you must look for an obvious deformity where the jaw meets the skull, check to see that the teeth line up, check to see if the athlete can move his jaw, and trace the jaw bone area to feel for bone chips or breaks in the bone. While making the visual and manual examination be aware of the below-mentioned injuries.

Treatment

Dislocation   A jaw dislocation results when the jaw bone is forced out of its jointure with the skull. This dislocation may be to just one side or to both sides at the same time resulting in a forward protrusion of the lower jaw so the teeth of the upper and lower jaws do not meet. There will be pain, and the athlete will not be able to move his jaw. Depending on the sport as well as the injury, the athlete will be disabled for up to three weeks.

A jaw dislocation is caused by a direct or glancing blow to the point of the chin or to the side of the jaw while the mouth is open, by a large yawn, or by the athlete taking too large a bite of food.

A jaw dislocation may be prevented by the athlete's wearing a mouth piece or a face guard. He should also use moderation in taking bites of food.

A jaw dislocation is treated with immediate application of cold packs and a bandage. In extreme emergencies *and only when it is impossible to get the athlete to a physician,* you may reduce the dislocation by wrapping both thumbs with gauze, then place your thumbs in his mouth so they rest on his teeth near the back of

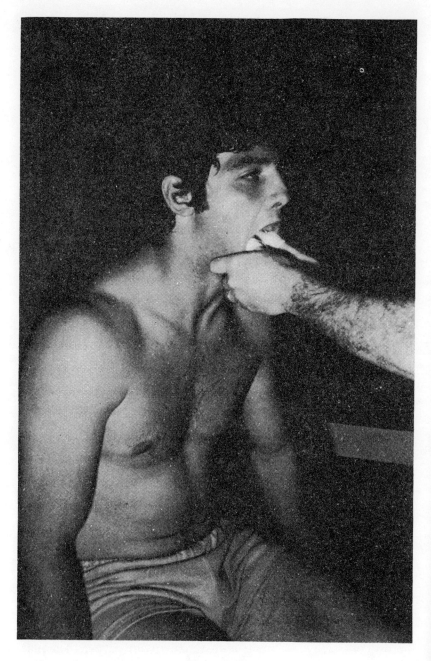

Figure 5-40

his mouth and your fingers are hooked under his chin. Press back and down with your thumbs while pulling forward and upward with your fingers (Figure 5-40). When his jaw starts in place, be sure to slip your thumbs out of his mouth so you will not be bitten. Should you decide to reduce the dislocation, it must be done immediately before the muscle contracts from pain and internal bleeding.

Jaw dislocation rehabilitation is under the supervision of the physician.

Fracture   A jaw fracture is a break of the upper jaw or cheekbone or the lower jaw. It is recognizable by the athlete's exhibiting an open mouth, drooling of saliva or blood, pain when jaw moves, and inability to line up his teeth.

A jaw fracture is caused by a blow to the point of the chin or to the jaw itself.

Jaw fracture may be prevented by the athlete's wearing a mouthguard and a face mask.

A jaw fracture is treated by closing the athlete's mouth so his upper and lower teeth are lined. Then secure the jaw with a bandage and transport the athlete to a physician.

Locked Jaw   A locked jaw is the inability of the athlete to open or close his mouth. It is usually painful and will frighten the athlete.

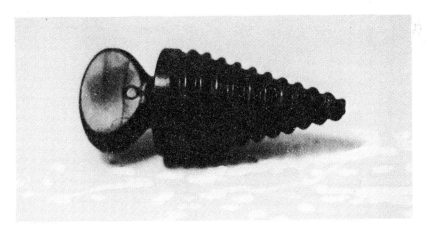

Figure 5-41

A locked jaw is caused by a blow to the jaw or the abdominal area, resulting in a muscle spasm.

A locked jaw may be prevented by the athlete's using a mouthguard or a face mask.

A locked jaw is treated by first making sure the athlete is breathing all right and his neck is not injured. Then place him in a face lying position and massage his jaw from in front of his ears to his chin. If this does not relax his jaw and his breathing becomes difficult, use an oral screw (Figure 5-41) to open his mouth.

Sprain   A jaw sprain occurs when the jaw is forced beyond its normal range of movement and results in damage to the muscles and ligaments. There will be pain but no loss of movement. The athlete may also have a slight variation in the alignment of his upper and lower teeth.

A jaw sprain is caused by the athlete's being hit on the chin or the jaw bone from a blow or a fall.

Jaw sprain may be prevented by the athlete's wearing a face mask and a mouthguard. He should also be instructed in proper techniques for protecting his face during competition.

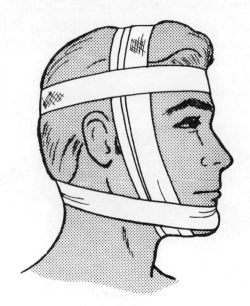

Figure 5-42

Strapping

Bandaging   Figure 5-42 illustrates a common technique for bandaging the jaw. This may be done with a wrap or tape, but the best material to use is a cloth bandage because it does not stretch or stick to the hair. Apply the bandage by rolling the cloth bandage into a roll. Then start the bandage on top of the athlete's head, go under his chin and then back to the top of his head. Continue until the roll is completely around his head and jaw. Next take a bandage and wrap it around the chin just below the mouth and around his neck. Finish by wrapping a bandage around the top of his head.

KNEE INJURIES

Anatomy

The knee is a hinge joint formed by the jointure of the upper leg bone (femur) with the big bone of the lower leg (tibia). This jointure is cushioned by the cartilage which is located between the upper and lower leg. It is stabilized by powerful ligaments, the outside (lateral), inside (medial), front (patellar), back (popliteal), and front and back cruciates. Along with these ligaments, there are the front (quadriceps) and back (hamstrings) thigh muscles and the calf (gastronemius and soleus) muscles.

Examination

When the knee is injured, look for obvious deformities, tender areas, limited range of motion, and point of injury. Point of injury may be determined with the following manual tests.

1. Figure 5-43 illustrates the bending and straightening test for determining cartilage damage. It is administered as follows: Have the athlete lie on his back. Then firmly grasp his lower leg and bend the knee as far as it will go. As soon as the athlete feels pain, tightness or blocking, stop and determine the locality of pain. Next apply gentle pressure and straighten the knee as far as pos-

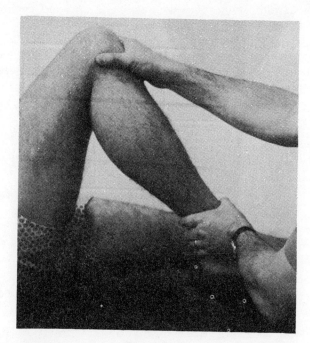

Figure 5-43

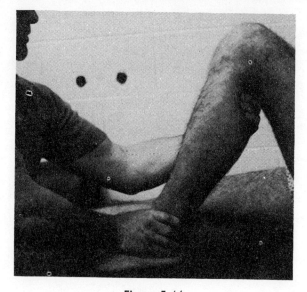

Figure 5-44

sible. Again, at the first point of pain, stop and determine the locality of the pain.

2. Figure 5-44 illustrates the front stability test for determining damage to the front cruciate ligament. It is administered as follows: Have the athlete lie on his back with his injured knee bent; grasp the foot of his injured knee and press downward in order to stabilize it. Then place your free hand behind the top part of the lower leg and pull away from his body.

3. Figure 5–45 illustrates the back stability test for determining damage to the back cruciate ligaments. It is administered as follows: Have the athlete lie on his back with his injured knee bent. Grasp his foot and apply slight downward pressure to keep it from moving. Then with your free hand placed at the top front of the lower leg push against the leg with slight pressure.

4. Figure 5-46 illustrates the side stability test for determining damage to side ligaments. It is administered as follows: Have the athlete lie on his back with his leg relaxed. Grasp his ankle and place your free hand on the outward side of his knee. Then move the lower leg from side to side. If there is an excessive amount of movement, it is a good practice to test both legs because the athlete may just have loose joints.

Treatment

After the knee examination has been completed, prompt and proper treatment must begin. Therefore, treatment procedures for bursitis, cartilage damage, contusion, cruciate ligament damage, dislocation, locked knee, Osgood-Schlatter fracture, side ligament damage, and water on the knee are knee injuries with which you should be familiar.

Bursitis   Knee bursitis is an inflammation of one or all of the bursae located on top of, back of, and below the kneecap. There will be localized heat, tenderness, and swelling in the area of the kneecap. Movement may be somewhat limited.

Knee bursitis is usually caused by a succession of minor bumps. However, severe twisting or hyperextension of the knee may cause damage to the bursae.

Knee bursitis is best prevented by immediate treatment of any bruise and protective pads for the area when the athlete participates.

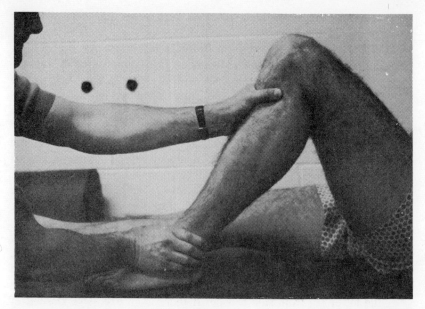

Figure 5-45

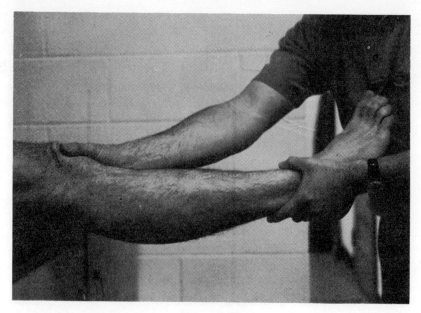

Figure 5-46

Knee bursitis is first treated with the application of an elastic wrap to reduce swelling and cold packs to reduce heat. Cold packs are frequently applied until all swelling has been reduced. At this time, heat, massage, and hot packs may be used. For extreme cases fluid may be drawn from the area by a physician.

Knee bursitis rehabilitation includes the use of heat, massage, hot packs, and mild exercise. This exercise has the athlete gently bending and straightening his knee so that the knee area is warmed before participation. Application of protective pads is necessary for participation (Figure 5-47).

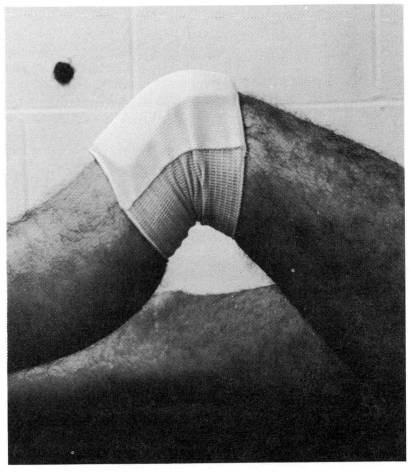

Figure 5-47

Cartilage Damage   The symptoms of a damaged cartilage
are leg fatigue, severe tenderness over the jointure of the upper and
lower legs, pain upon movement, localized swelling, and limitation
of movement. In some cases, cartilage damage can be felt, as well
as heard, when your hand is placed on the jointure of the knee with
the big bone of the lower leg (Figure 5-48). When the lower leg is
moved, a click can be felt and sometimes heard.

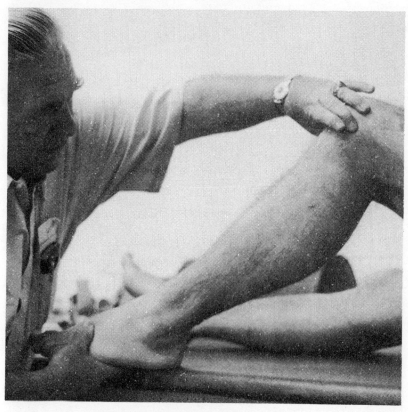

Figure 5-48

Cartilage damage is caused by a violent, forceful inward or
outward turning of the upper leg bone on the big bone of the lower
leg.

Cartilage damage treatment begins with gentle application of
an elastic wrap, cold packs, and elevation of the knee above the
head. Care must be taken to keep the leg from bending while treatment is in progress. Next day apply heat, massage, and hot packs.

Use muscle setting exercises for strengthening the quadriceps.

Cartilage damage rehabilitative procedures include frequent use of heat, massage, hot packs, and exercises. As soon as soreness is diminished and a physician gives an okay, the area is stretched by having the athlete slowly bend and then straighten his knee.

Contusion   Knee contusion is very common in athletics because the muscles of the knee joint are near the bone and thus can easily be damaged by a blow. Swelling of the area is immediate and severe.

Knee contusion is caused by a violent blow to the knee which forces the muscles against the bone.

Knee contusion may be prevented by the use of protective knee pads.

Knee contusion is treated with immediate application of cold packs and an elastic wrap. Next day apply heat, massage, and hot packs.

Knee contusion rehabilitative procedures include the use of heat, massage, hot packs, and exercises.

Cruciate Ligament Damage   Cruciate ligaments hold the lower leg bones in place at the jointure of the knee. Symptoms of damage to the cruciates include pain, loss of function, knee fatigue, tenderness, and swelling.

Cruciate ligament damage is caused by an excessive bending of the knee too far backward (hyperextension). The usual force is a severe twisting.

Cruciate ligament damage may be prevented with stretching and strengthening exercises for the upper thighs and lower legs.

Cruciate ligament damage treatment includes cold packs, elastic wrap, and elevation of the knee above the head. Be sure that the leg remains straight throughout the treatment, and follow up by having a physician check the injured area.

Cruciate ligament damage rehabilitative procedures include the daily use of heat, massage, hot packs, and exercises.

Dislocation   A knee dislocation most frequently involves the kneecap or lower leg bones. There will be cartilage, ligament, and bursae damage. Deformity, loss of movement, and swelling will also be present.

Kneecap dislocation is caused by a severe blow when the

athlete falls or is hit. Lower leg bone dislocation is caused by a severe twist of the lower leg.

Knee dislocation may be prevented with stretching and strengthening exercises of the upper and lower leg muscles.

Knee dislocation treatment includes application of cold packs, elastic wrap, and a splint. Then the athlete is transported to the physician for further treatment.

Knee dislocation rehabilitation is carried out under a physician's supervision.

Locked Knee   Locked knee results when the cartilage is broken and part of it becomes lodged in the knee joint. Usually, there will be swelling and loss of movement.

Locked knee is caused by a violent, forceful inward or outward turning of the upper leg bone on the big bone of the lower leg.

Locked knee may be prevented by having the athlete use frequent strengthening exercises for the upper and lower legs.

Locked knee treatment includes cold packs, an elastic wrap, and elevation of the knee above the head. Next day have the athlete sit on a table with his legs hanging downward. Then have him swing his lower leg back and forth and twist it from side to side.

Locked knee rehabilitation utilizes daily heat, massage, hot packs, and exercise.

Osgood-Schlatter Fracture   The Osgood-Schlatter fracture is not a break, but instead it is a partial outward separation of the big bone of the lower leg from the lower jointure of the knee. There will be pain upon bending and kneeling, and an abnormal lump with local tenderness is noticeable just below the kneecap. The athlete will often walk stiff-legged to ease the pain. This type of fracture is more prevalent among junior and senior high school students because the head of the bone of the lower leg has not become hardened.

Osgood-Schlatter fracture is caused by a twisting or a sharp blow which results in a partial separation of the lower leg bone from the joint.

Osgood-Schlatter fracture treatment includes cold packs and an elastic wrap. For severe cases, apply a splint and transport the athlete to a physician. Heat, massage, and hot packs help speed recovery.

Osgood-Schlatter fracture rehabilitation includes close supervision of the physician as well as the frequent use of heat.

Side Ligament Damage   The ligaments on each side of the knee joint furnish stabilization, and when these ligaments are stretched or torn, there will be localized swelling and tenderness, loss of movement, and severe pain on bending or straightening the knee.

Side ligament damage is caused when the knee is severely twisted or there is an outward or inward forcing caused by a sharp blow. The inside ligament (medial) is most frequently injured by a blow on the outside of the knee.

Side ligament damage is hard to prevent, but probably the best method is to strengthen the front and back thigh muscles and lower leg muscles so that the knee will be more stable.

Side ligament damage treatment includes application of cold packs and compression bandage to prevent swelling. Next day, if the athlete is able to move his knee without undue pain, apply heat, massage, and hot packs.

Side ligament damage rehabilitation includes frequent use of heat, massage, hot packs, and exercise.

Water on the Knee   Water on the knee is an inflammation of the membrane which covers the ends of the upper and lower leg bones at their jointure.

Water on the knee is caused by repeated blows or a severe blow to the knee joint.

Water on the knee may be prevented with knee pads.

Water on the knee is treated with cold packs, elastic wrap, and elevation of the knee above the head. As soon as possible, usually the next day, apply heat, massage, and hot packs to the knee.

Water on the knee rehabilitation is the same as treatment with the exception of rest until the swelling subsides. At this time begin exercises.

Exercises

Isometric and *isotonic* exercises for the knee are performed according to the directions on page 44.

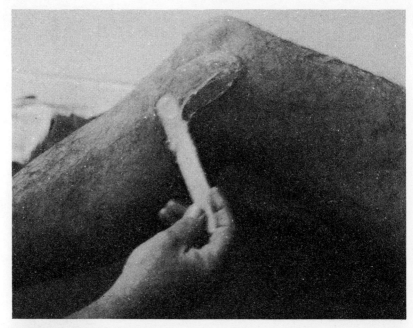

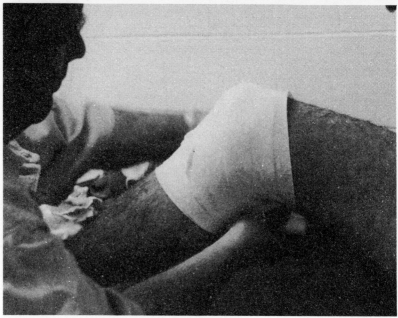

Figure 5-49

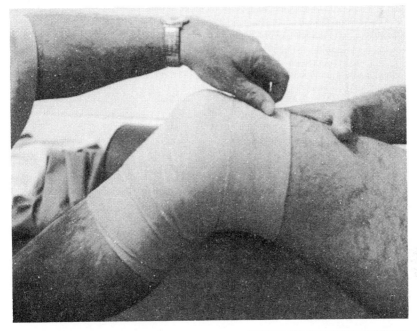

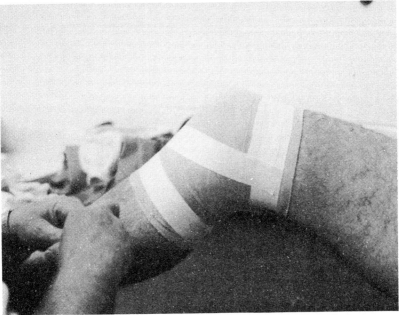

Figure 5-49 continued

Strapping

After the knee has been treated and exercised, it must then be protected with either a hot pack or tape.

Hot Pack   The knee hot pack provides warmth to the injured area. It is made by applying analgesic balm, covering with cotton, and securing with an elastic wrap (Figure 5-49). Hot packs are usually continued until the knee is completely rehabilitated.

Taping   Before applying tape to the athlete's knee, be sure that his knee area is clean, dry, and free of hair. Then have the athlete stand with his knee slightly bent. Apply anchor strips (see #1 in Figure 5-50) just above and below the knee cap. Then bring a vertical strip of tape from the bottom anchor up over the top of the leg and attach to the top anchor on the opposite side of the leg (see #2 in Figure 5-50). Continue taping until the knee area is covered. Complete the taping job by putting an elastic wrap around the entire taped area.

SHOULDER INJURIES

Anatomy

The shoulder is a ball and socket joint which includes the collar bone (clavicle), shoulder blade (scapula), breast bone (sternum), and upper arm bone (humerus). These bones are held together by muscles, ligaments, and tendons. There are three joints in the shoulder area with which you must become familiar. These are the shoulder joint formed by the upper arm bone and the shoulder blade, the acromio-clavicular joint formed by the collar bone and acromion process, and the sterno-clavicular joint formed by the collar bone and breast bone.

Examination

Whenever a shoulder injury occurs, you must first learn how the athlete was injured. As soon as you have this needed informa-

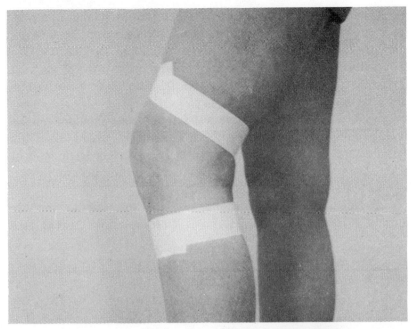

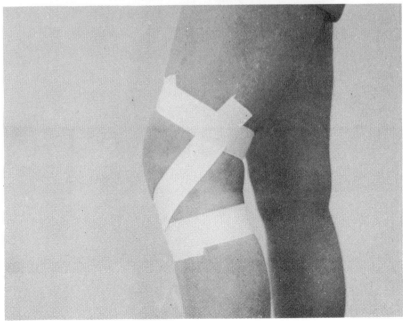

Figure 5-50

tion, you inspect the area for obvious deformities, tender areas, and for loss of movement. During the stage of inspection, be sure you compare the injured shoulder with the uninjured shoulder to see if they differ. Be sure to feel the area around each of the three joints to check for dislocations or possible fractures before performing the following tests for point of injury.

Figure 5-51 illustrates the test for the front shoulder muscle. It is administered as follows: With the athlete seated, have him raise his arm in front of his body so it forms a right angle with his body. Then grasp his arm and have him try to raise his arm upward against your light downward pressure.

Figure 5-52 illustrates the test for the middle shoulder muscle. It is administered as follows: With the athlete seated, have

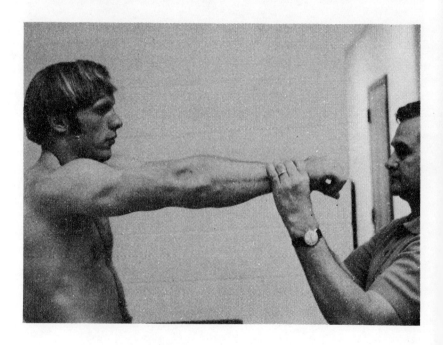

Figure 5-51

him raise his arm out at his side so it forms a right angle with his body. Grasp his arm and apply slight downward pressure as he tries to raise his arm.

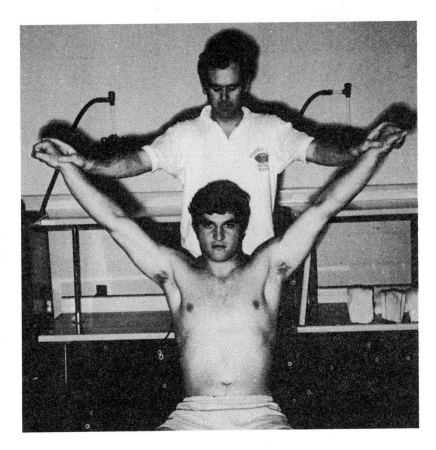

Figure 5-52

The test for the back shoulder muscle is administered as follows: With the athlete lying face down, have him raise his arm upward and lock his elbow. Apply slight downward pressure on his arm as he tries to move his arm upward away from his body (Figure 4-8).

The test for the upper shoulder muscles is administered as follows: Have the athlete lie face down with arms palms up at his sides. Place one hand on his upper back and one hand on the back

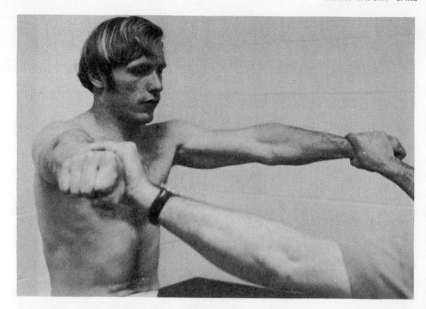

Figure 5-53

of his head and have him raise his head upward against the pressure (Figure 4-7).

Figure 5-53 illustrates the test for the chest muscles. It is administered as follows: Have the athlete sit on a table and raise his arm so it forms a right angle with his body. Apply pressure on his arm, above the elbow, as he tries to bring his arm across his body.

Treatment

As soon as the shoulder examination has been completed, prompt and proper treatment begins. Therefore, you must be familiar with treatment procedures for bursitis, contusion, dislocation, fracture, separation, and sprain.

Bursitis   Shoulder bursitis affects the shoulder joint where the upper arm bone and shoulder blade meet. It is an inflammation of the bursae and will be painful and limit movement. The athlete will not be able to touch the small of his back, and the shoulder area may be warm to the touch.

Shoulder bursitis is usually caused by a hard blow to or severe twisting of the shoulder joint causing the bursae to swell and exert pressure inside the joint.

Shoulder bursitis may be prevented by wearing shoulder pads or other protective pads.

Shoulder bursitis is treated by application of cold and a sling. Next day apply hot and cold treatments and provide a sling.

Shoulder bursitis is rehabilitated by following treatment procedure until all pain has diminished and there is free movement in the shoulder joint. Then and only then do you start exercises.

Contusion   A shoulder contusion is a bruise to the muscle of the shoulder area. The most common shoulder contusion is to the acromion process. These shoulder contusions are very painful and will in some cases cause restriction of movement. There will also be discoloration and swelling. In localized contusion the athlete will so indicate by pointing to the area, and in generalized contusion he will use his whole hand to show you the injury.

A shoulder contusion is caused by a sharp blow to the shoulder when the athlete falls or is tackled.

Shoulder contusion may be prevented by wearing shoulder pads which fit and by teaching proper fundamentals of tackling.

A shoulder contusion is treated by immediate application of cold and a compression bandage to prevent swelling. Next day apply heat, massage, and hot packs.

A shoulder contusion is rehabilitated by continuous use of heat, massage, and exercise. For the acromion process contusion, you must apply a sponge rubber or felt pad which has a hole slightly larger than the contused area. Tape this to the shoulder before the athlete puts on his shoulder pads or before he participates (Figure 5-54).

Dislocation   A shoulder dislocation is a complete displacement of the upper arm bone from its jointure with the shoulder blade. There will be pain, swelling, loss of movement, and a definite deformity.

A shoulder dislocation is caused by a twisting of the joints past their normal range of motion as a result of falls, blows, or twists of the arm.

A shoulder dislocation may be prevented by wearing proper protective gear and strengthening and stretching exercises.

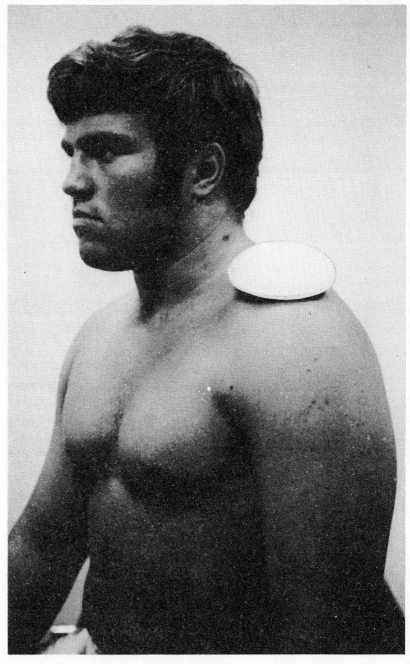

Figure 5-54

A shoulder dislocation is treated by the physician who makes the reduction. However, you may apply cold to the area to reduce swelling and a sling to prevent further internal damage. Transport the athlete to the physician as quickly as possible.

A shoulder dislocation rehabilitation proceeds under the physician's care. When the physician releases the athlete, use heat, massage, hot packs, and exercises. For competition, you may use a shoulder harness to prevent the shoulder from going past a predetermined range of motion (Figure 5-55).

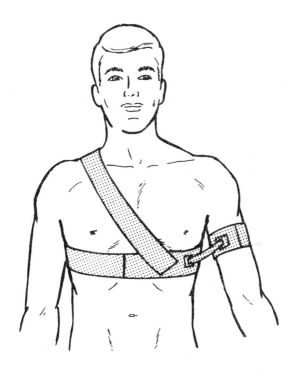

Figure 5-55

Fracture   A shoulder fracture is a break of one or more of the bones which make up the shoulder. The most common shoulder fracture is a break of the collar bone. In most cases the fracture will be apparent, but in other instances you might need to have the shoulder X-rayed to determine the point and extent of the fracture.

There will be pain, swelling, deformity, and loss of movement. Always be aware of and prepare for treatment of open wounds since the broken bones sometimes break through the skin.

A shoulder fracture is caused by blows to the shoulder area or by the athlete's falling on his shoulder.

A shoulder fracture may be prevented by wearing protective padding and by teaching of proper falling and tackling techniques.

A shoulder fracture is treated by immediate immobilization of the joint, application of a sling, and transportation to the physician who will set the shoulder. You may during the trip to the physician keep cold packs on the area to prevent swelling and to reduce pain.

A shoulder fracture rehabilitation proceeds under the physician's supervision.

Separation   A shoulder separation is the partial dislocation of one of the shoulder bones from its jointure. There will be pain and partial loss of movement because of swelling and damage to muscle tissue around the joint. The most common shoulder separations occur at the acromio-clavicular joint and the sterno-clavicular joint.

A shoulder separation is caused by a twist of the joint or by the athlete's falling on the point of his shoulder or on his outstretched arm. Sometimes a separation results from a hard blow to one of the bones in the shoulder area.

Shoulder separation may be prevented by strengthening and stretching exercises and wearing of proper protective padding.

A shoulder separation is treated with an immediate application of cold and a compression bandage. Next day apply heat, massage, and hot packs.

Shoulder separation rehabilitation includes use of heat, massage, hot packs, and exercises to prevent atrophy (wasting away) of the muscles. Be sure to provide enough protective padding to prevent reinjury to the separated area.

Sprain   A shoulder sprain occurs when the shoulder joint (upper arm bone and shoulder blade) is forced beyond its normal range of motion. There will be intense pain, swelling, and limitation of movement. However, there will be no major deformity at the jointure. Usually there will be some swelling in the immediate area of the sprain.

A shoulder sprain is caused by a twisting or jerking of the arm past the joint's normal range.

A shoulder sprain may be prevented with strengthening and stretching exercises.

A shoulder sprain is treated with cold packs and a compression bandage. Next day apply heat, massage, hot packs, and exercise.

A shoulder sprain is rehabilitated with continued use of heat, massage, and exercise. For practice and games, apply tape or wrap to prevent re-injury of the joint. In questionable cases, use a shoulder harness to reduce the chances of the shoulder joint's being forced out of its socket.

Exercises

Following is a description of isometric and isotonic exercises for strengthening the shoulder muscles.

Isometric Exercises   Each of the following isometric exercises is done for eight seconds twice daily.

The exercise for strengthening the front shoulder muscle is administered as follows: With the athlete seated, have him raise his arm in front of his body so it forms a right angle with his body. Then apply downward pressure as he tries to raise his arm upward (Figure 5-51).

The exercise for strengthening the middle shoulder muscle is administered as follows: With the athlete seated, have him raise his arm out at his side so it forms a right angle with his upper body. Then apply downward pressure as he tries to raise his arm upward (Figure 5-52).

The exercise for strengthening the back shoulder muscle is administered as follows: With the athlete lying face down, have him raise his arm upward and lock his elbow. Then apply downward pressure on his wrist as he tries to raise his arm. (Figure 4-8).

The exercise for strengthening the upper shoulder muscles is administered as follows: Have the athlete lie face down with arms palms up at his sides. Place one hand on the back of his head and one hand on his upper back. Then have him try to raise his head upward against the downward pressure (Figure 4-7).

The exercise for strengthening the chest muscles is administered as follows: With the athlete seated, have him raise his arm so it forms a right angle with his body. Then apply outward pressure against his arm as he tries to bring his arm across his body (Figure 5-53).

Figure 5-56 illustrates the exercise for strengthening the muscles which rotate the arm at the shoulder joint. It is administered as follows: With the athlete seated, have him raise his arm out at his side so it forms a right angle with his body. Then grasp his hand and have him rotate his arm against your resistance. For best results, he should rotate both ways.

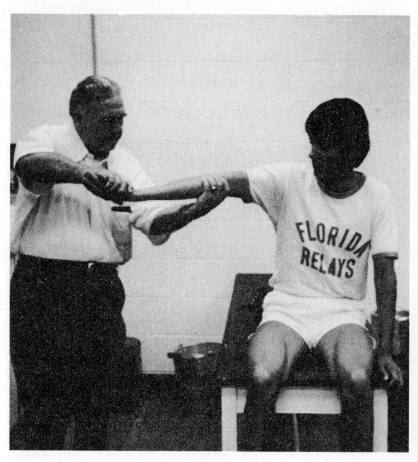

Figure 5-56

Isotonic Exercises   Each of the following isotonic exercises are performed according to the directions described on page 65.

Figure 5-57 illustrates the exercise for strengthening the front shoulder muscles. It is administered as follows: With the athlete seated, have him grasp a weight, turn his palm down, and bring his

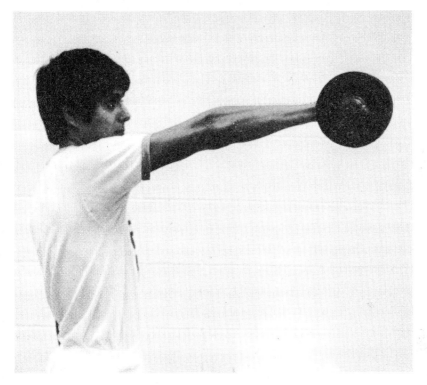

Figure 5-57

arm down at his side. Next he should bring the weight up so that his arm forms a right angle with his upper body and then return the weight to the starting position.

Figure 5-58 illustrates the exercise for the middle shoulder muscle. It is administered as follows: With the athlete seated, have him grasp a weight, turn his palm down, and bring his arm to his side. Next he should raise his arm so that it forms a right angle with his body and then return the weight to its starting position.

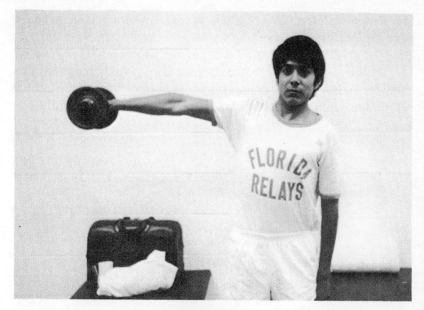

Figure 5-58

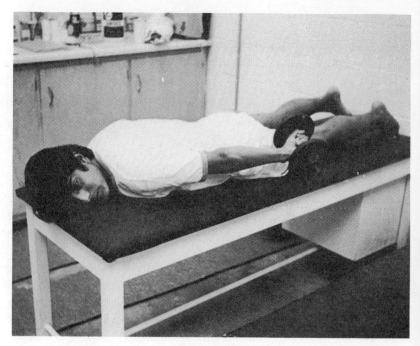

Figure 5-59

Figure 5-59 illustrates the exercise for strengthening the back shoulder muscle. It is administered as follows: With the athlete lying face down, have him grasp a weight and turn his thumb up. Next he should move his arm upward as high as possible and then return it to its starting position.

Figure 5-60 illustrates the exercise for stretching the shoulder muscles. It is administered as follows: With the athlete standing erect, have him place his right arm over his right shoulder and bring his left arm up behind his back and grasp his right hand. Repeat the same procedure with the left arm over the left shoulder. *If the athlete cannot do this, have him reach his arms as high as possible or else have him hang by his hands from a bar for ten seconds.*

Strapping

Hot Pack The shoulder hot pack is applied by placing a thin coating of analgesic balm on the injured area, covering with a layer of cotton, and wrapping with an elastic wrap.

Wrapping The shoulder wrap is applied by starting the wrap twice around the athlete's upper arm, going across his back, around his neck, and back under his arm. Continue until the wrap has been exhausted (Figure 5-61).

Taping The particular tape technique will depend on the site of the injury.

Figure 5-62 illustrates a tape technique useful for most shoulder injuries. It is applied as follows: Have the athlete stand with his elbow bent and his wrist held by his other hand. Then spray the area to be taped with skin toughener. Next apply a strip of tape from an area between the breasts, alongside the neck, and down to a point below the shoulder blade. Cover the breast with a gauze pad. Then bring a piece of tape from the front of the body beginning at the lower end of the first strip of tape around the arm to the end of the first strip of tape on the athlete's back. Alternately apply the vertical and horizontal strips until the entire shoulder area has been covered with tape.

Figure 5-63 illustrates a tape technique for a sternoclavicular sprain or separation. It is administered as follows: Have the athlete stand. Cover his breast with a gauze pad and then spray the area to

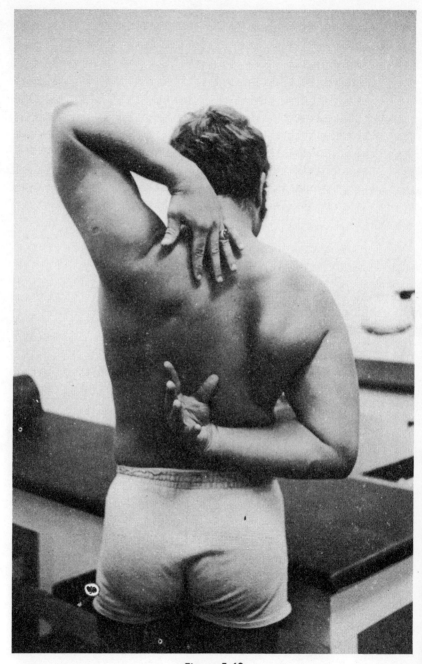

Figure 5-60

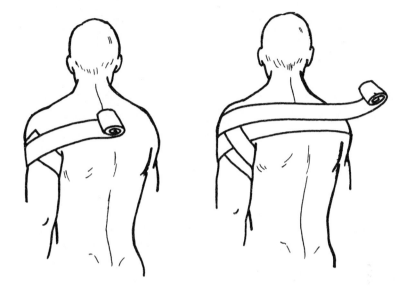

Figure 5-61

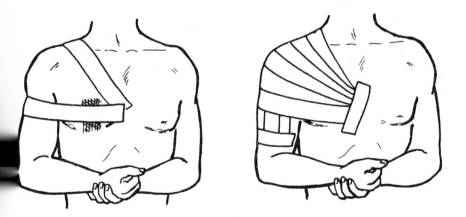

Figure 5-62

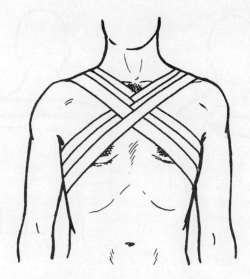

Figure 5-63

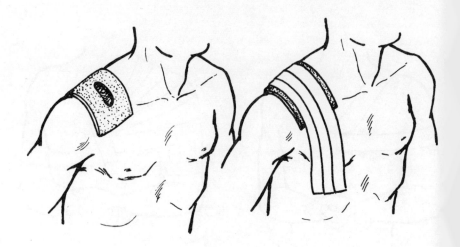

Figure 5-64

be taped with skin toughener. Anchor a piece of tape below the shoulder blade, bring it up around his neck, and down under his arm and anchor approximately six inches on his back. Continue the same procedure with four or five strips of tape in such a way they overlap each other. Next anchor the ends of the long strips with a piece of tape to prevent the tape from curling.

Figure 5-64 illustrates the tape technique for the acromio-clavicular separation or sprain. It is administered as follows: Have the athlete stand with his elbow bent and supported by his other hand. Cover his breast with a gauze pad. Next place a piece of felt over the acromio-clavicular joint. Spray the area to be taped with skin toughener. Start the first strip of tape at a point just below the shoulder blade and come over the acromio-clavicular joint down to a point just below the breast. The second strip of tape is started at the front and goes over to the back. Alternately apply five or six strips of tape in an overlapping manner.

WRIST INJURIES

Anatomy

The wrist is a gliding joint formed by the jointure of the lower end of the lower arm bones with the eight wrist bones. It is held together by ligaments, and its movements are effected by the tendons of the muscles of the lower arm.

Examination

Whenever a wrist injury occurs, you must first learn how the injury happened. Determine the position of the athlete's wrist at the time of the injury, whether the athlete heard anything, and whether the athlete felt any particular sensation. Pay particular attention to the position of the wrist when the athlete reported the injury to you. Next compare both wrists to see if they differ. Then feel the wrist area by starting with the forearm, wrist, and hand bones. If you detect no obvious fractures or dislocations, have the athlete move his hand up at the wrist, down at the wrist, inward at the wrist, outward at the wrist, and rotate the hand at the wrist.

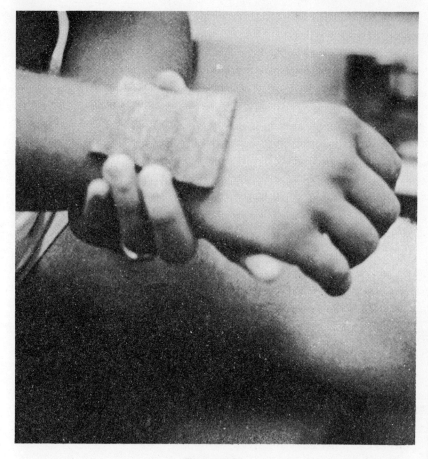

Figure 5-65

Treatment

After completing the examination of the wrist area, concentrate on treating one of the following injuries.

Contusion   A wrist contusion is a bruise to the wrist area resulting in discoloration, soreness, and rapid swelling. Usually the athlete will experience severe pain only when the contused area is hit.

A wrist contusion is caused by a blow to the wrist area or by the wrist's being stepped on.

A wrist contusion may be prevented by wearing padding over the wrist and hand area whenever there is a possibility of the athlete's hitting a hard surface or being hit by another player.

A wrist contusion is treated by an immediate application of cold, a compression bandage, and elevation to reduce swelling. Start heat treatments when swelling has ceased. Ordinarily swelling will have reached its peak within 24 to 48 hours after the wrist is injured. You may then start heat treatments and exercises.

A wrist contusion rehabilitation is started when there is no pain on movement and includes, besides heat, exercises for strengthening the area along with stretching of the wrist area through full range of movement. Be sure to keep the area covered with a hot pack and provide a sponge rubber pad or felt pad over the area when the athlete participates (Figure 5-65).

Dislocation   A wrist dislocation involves a displacement of one or more of the bones at the jointure of the wrist. The most common is the displacement of one of the arm bones from its articulation with the wrist bone. There will be an obvious deformity, swelling, loss of movement, muscle spasm, and severe pain in the vicinity of the wrist joint.

A wrist dislocation is caused by the athlete's falling so that his wrist is forced beyond its normal range of motion or else the wrist is severely twisted past its normal limits.

A wrist dislocation may be prevented by strengthening exercises and by teaching proper falling techniques. The athlete should be instructed to bring his arms toward his body when he falls.

A wrist dislocation is treated with immediate application of a splint and transportation of the athlete to a physician who will reduce the dislocation. You must not attempt to reduce the dislocation since there is usually a strong possibility of a fracture associated with the dislocation.

Wrist dislocation rehabilitation is under the physician's supervision.

Fracture   A wrist fracture usually involves the lower end of the two arm bones or the wrist bone which joins the arm bones. The first is called Colles' fracture (Figure 5-66) and the second is called a navicular fracture (Figure 5-67). There will be pain on movement, swelling, and loss of movement in the wrist area. You may be able to feel the break by gently pressing the wrist area where the lower arm bones articulate with the wrist bones. You may detect the navicular fracture by feeling the wrist area between the large bone of the lower arm and the thumb.

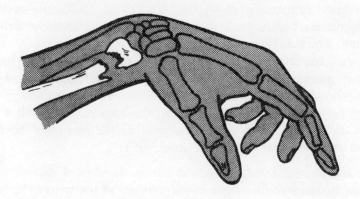

Figure 5-66

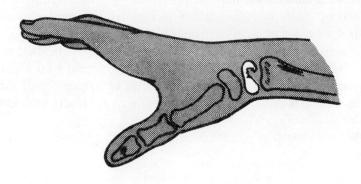

Figure 5-67

A Colles' fracture is caused by a blow to the wrist area or by the athlete's falling on his outstretched hand. The navicular fracture is most generally caused by the athlete's falling on his outstretched hand. However, there have been rare cases of its being broken by a blow.

A wrist fracture may be prevented by strengthening exercises and protective padding on the wrist in contact sports. Falling techniques will also help.

A wrist fracture is treated with application of a splint and transportation to the physician. You might apply cold to the area while in transit to prevent excessive swelling.

A wrist fracture rehabilitation is under the physician's supervision.

Ganglion A wrist ganglion is a herniation of the tendon sheath or joint covering (capsule) which becomes filled with a clear fluid causing a bulge on the wrist. This bulge usually appears on the top of the wrist but it can appear other places (Figure 5-68).

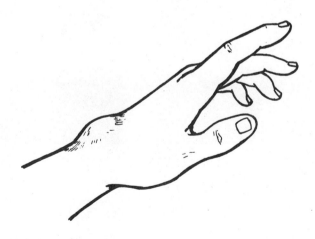

Figure 5-68

A wrist ganglion is caused by a blow to the wrist severe enough to break the tendon sheath. Repeated blows to an untreated wrist will also contribute to the ganglion.

A wrist ganglion may be prevented by wearing protective padding over the wrist area and by immediately treating any bruised area on the wrist.

A wrist ganglion is treated by application of a felt pad on the ganglion and a compression bandage as illustrated in Figure 5-69. The best method is surgery to correct the tear in the tendon sheath. The area might be aspirated (fluid drawn off with a needle) by the team physician.

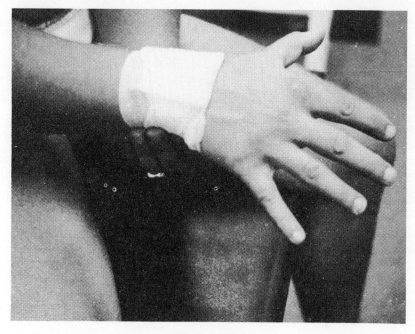

Figure 5-69

A wrist ganglion is rehabilitated by the surgical removal of the problem by the physician. Start rehabilitative exercises as soon as the physician will permit them.

Sprain   A wrist sprain is a stretching or tearing of the ligaments, tendons and tissue around the wrist joint. There will be pain, swelling, and some loss of movement. Severe sprains might cause complete loss of movement and appearance of a slight knot on the wrist.

A wrist sprain is caused by the athlete's falling on his bent wrist or by the athlete's hand being violently twisted at the wrist.

A wrist sprain may be prevented by strengthening the forearm muscles and by teaching proper falling techniques. Some coaches and trainers advocate the taping of the wrist or wearing a leather wrist support to prevent sprains; however, I feel that the strengthening exercises are much better.

A wrist sprain is treated by first making an exact determination of its degree of severity. When there is an inability of the athlete to move his hand upward toward his arm and generalized swelling, treat the sprain as a fracture by immobilizing it with a splint and transporting the athlete to a physician so an X ray can be made. For those sprains in which there is moderate pain on movement and light swelling, apply cold packs and a compression bandage. Next day use heat, hot packs, and hand exercises.

A wrist sprain rehabilitation is a follow-up of heat, hot packs, and exercises. For practice and games be sure to tape the area so that it cannot move past a predetermined range of motion. Rehabilitation of the wrist will take at least a week or more before it is completely healed. Therefore, you must adhere to treatment procedures daily regardless of the athlete's reluctance to have the wrist treated.

Exercises

Following are isometric and isotonic exercises for wrist injury rehabilitation.

Isometric Exercises   Each of the following exercises is done for eight seconds twice daily.

1. Figure 5-70 illustrates the upward movement exercise which is administered as follows: Have the athlete turn his palm down and bend his wrist so that his fingers are pointed down. You then grasp his arm just above his wrist with one hand and place your other hand on top of his hand. Apply slight pressure against his upward movement.
2. Figure 5-71 illustrates the downward movement exercise which is administered as follows: Have the athlete turn his palm down

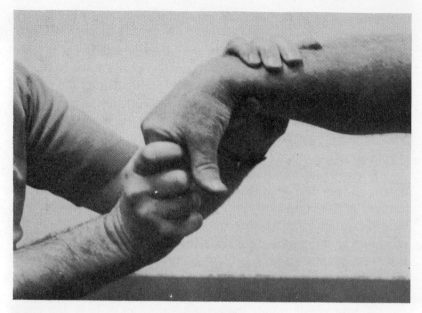

Figure 5-70

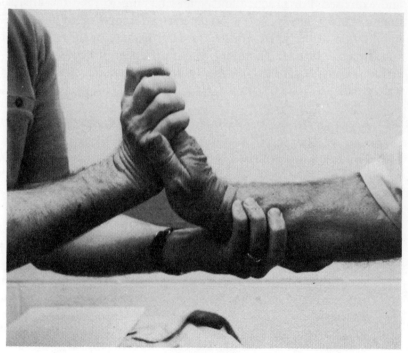

Figure 5-71

and bend his wrist so that his fingers are pointed upward. Then you grasp his arm just above his wrist with one hand and place your other hand in his palm. Apply slight pressure against his upward movement.

3. Figure 5-72 illustrates the inward movement exercise which is administered as follows: Have the athlete turn his palm down and straighten his wrist. Grasp his arm just above his wrist with one hand and place your other hand on the thumb side of his hand. Then have him turn his hand outward as far as possible. While his hand is in this position, apply pressure as he tries to turn his hand back to the inside.

4. Figure 5-73 illustrates the outward movement exercise which is administered as follows: Have the athlete turn his palm down and straighten his wrist. Grasp his arm just above his wrist with one hand and place your other hand on the little finger side of his hand. Then have him turn his hand inward as far as possible. While his hand is in this position, apply pressure as he tries to turn his hand back to the outside.

Isotonic Exercises   Each of the following isotonic exercises are performed according to the directions described on page 65.

1. Figure 5-74 illustrates the exercise for the muscles which rotate the wrist. It is administered as follows: Have the athlete stand with his lower arm at a right angle to his upper body. Next have him grasp a weight and turn his thumb up. From this starting position he turns the weight all the way to his right and all the way to his left.

2. The exercise for the muscles which move the hand up at the wrist is administered as follows: The athlete is seated so that his wrist extends over the edge of a table. He grasps a weight and turns his palm down. From this position he raises the weight as high as possible and returns it to the starting position without lifting his arm.

3. The exercise for the muscles which move the hand down at the wrist is administered as follows: The athlete is seated as described above. He grasps a weight and turns his palm up. From this position he raises the weight as high as possible and returns to the starting position.

4. Figure 5-75 illustrates the exercise for the muscles which assist in the grasping of the hand. It is administered by having the athlete stand. Then have him hold the bar attached to the weighted line. Next have him roll the weight all the way up to the rod and then roll the weight back down.

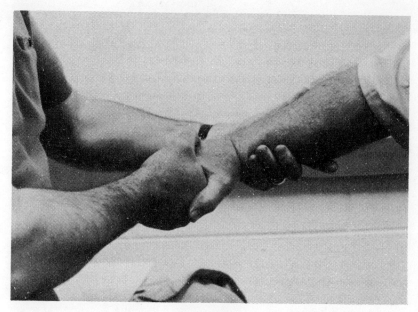

Figure 5-72

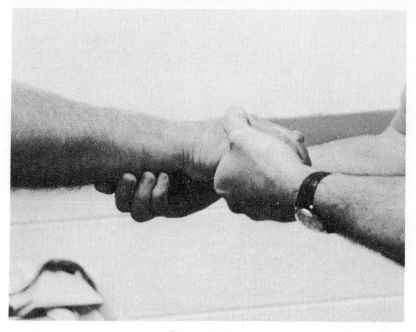

Figure 5-73

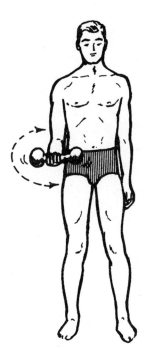

Figure 5-74

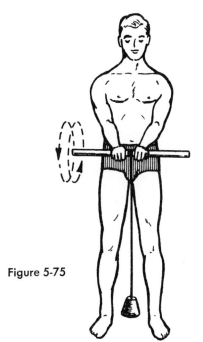

Figure 5-75

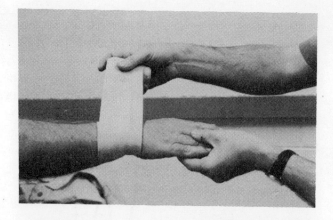

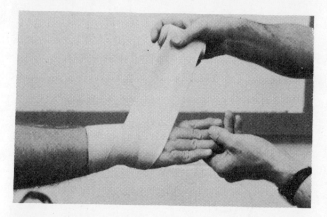

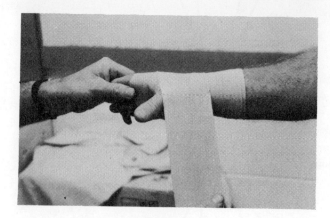

Figure 5-76

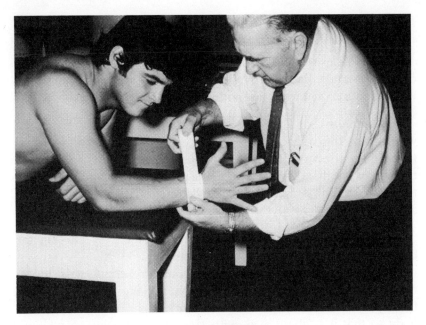

Figure 5-77

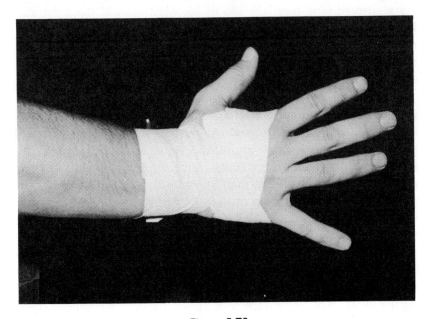

Figure 5-78

Strapping

Hot Pack   The wrist hot pack is applied by putting a thin coating of analgesic balm over the wrist area, covering with a thin layer of cotton, and wrapping with an elastic wrap.

Wrapping   The wrist wrap is done with a narrow elastic wrap. Start the wrap on top of the wrist and go around several times in the direction of thumb to fingers. Then take the wrap across the top of the hand, around underneath the palm, and across between the thumb and index finger back over the wrist. Continue around the wrist until all the wrap is used (Figure 5-76).

Taping   The wrist is prepared for taping by shaving the hair and spraying the area with skin toughener.

Figure 5-77 shows the tape technique for limiting wrist movement. It is applied as follows: Have the athlete stand so that he faces you. Then have him raise his arm straight out in front of his body so that it is about even with your lower rib cage. Next have him spread his fingers as far apart as possible. In this position, apply a strip of tape from the top of his wrist around the wrist and back to the top of his wrist. Apply five or six more strips of tape so that they overlap each other about half-way. Be sure you make the tape snug, not tight, and tape from the bottom of the arm upward and apply only one strip at a time.

Figure 5-78 shows the tape technique for restricting wrist movements. It is administered as follows: The athlete assumes the same position described above. Apply two anchor strips, one approximately three inches above the wrist and one around the knuckles of the hand. Next apply a strip of tape from the bottom anchor to the top anchor so that it crosses the wrist at an angle. Do the same with another strip of tape so that when it is in place the two strips of tape form an "X" on the wrist area. Apply these strips of tape in an overlapping manner across the back of the hand until the entire area is covered. Then enclose the wrist and hand with circular strips of tape. The amount of tape you use will depend on the degree of the injury and the amount of movement you are going to allow. The more tape you apply, the less movement there will be. Be certain the tape is not tight enough to cut off circulation.

6

Head Injury Care

The head is formed by the fusion of the eight cranial and fourteen facial bones. It can, for athletic training purposes, be divided into three regions, the brain, face, and scalp. Head injuries are complex and may, if not properly and immediately handled, develop into a serious condition. Common sites of head injuries include the brain, ear, eye, face, mouth, nose, scalp, and skull.

BRAIN INJURIES

A brain injury is serious and will present you with a perplexing problem. It varies from a mild headache to coma. Regardless of the degree of injury immediate attention is a must. Symptoms of brain injury include blurred vision, bleeding from ears, convulsion, disorientation, dilated eye pupils, headache, loss of memory, nausea, unconsciousness, paralysis, and vomiting. The most common brain injury with which you must become familiar is the concussion.

Concussion

A brain concussion is a jarring or shaking of the brain. Its symptoms vary, but basically the athlete may be dizzy, feel faint, be drowsy, have a headache, have labored breathing, have a loss of strength, have an unsteady pulse, and have unequal eye pupils which do not react to light.

A brain concussion is caused by a blow to the face, chin, or head. The athlete may experience a concussion from falling or sitting down very hard.

A brain concussion may be prevented by wearing properly fitted headgear, face masks, and mouth guards.

A brain concussion must have immediate treatment. First, check to be sure that air passages are open. Then use a small dose of smelling salts to help the athlete regain consciousness. Check for coherence by asking the athlete simple questions. Next test his strength by having the athlete squeeze your hand. Finally, check his eye reaction to light. When the athlete does not appear normal, place him on a stretcher and transport him to a physician for observation. Never let an athlete re-enter a contest after he has been knocked unconscious until he has been checked by the physician.

A brain concussion rehabilitation is under the physician's supervision.

EAR INJURIES

The ear is divided into three parts, the internal, middle, and external. You need only concern yourself with external and middle ear injuries. Ear injuries with which you must be familiar follow:

Cauliflower

Cauliflower ear is a swelling and accumulation of solidified blood or fluid between the skin and cartilage. It will be painful, swollen, discolored, tender, and numb. It is also unsightly.

Cauliflower ear is caused by a blow, repeated rubbing, or twisting of headgear on the ear.

Cauliflower ear may be prevented by wearing headgear which fits or by rubbing a skin lubricant on the ear. Potential cauliflower ear can be prevented by applying cold on the ear when it becomes hot from excessive rubbing as in wrestling.

Cauliflower ear is treated with an immediate application of cold and a compression bandage for thirty minutes or more. If a blood formation in the form of a bulge appears, send the athlete to the team physician.

Cauliflower ear is rehabilitated with cold packs and compression bandage. Figure 6-1 shows you how to apply a compression bandage to the ear. Place gauze pads or a piece of cotton under the edge of the top of the ear and between the ear and the head. Then cover with an elastic wrap. This procedure should be followed for at least a week, and when the athlete participates, provide protection for the ear.

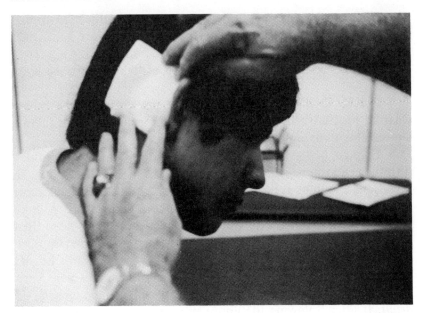

Figure 6-1

Cut (Tear)

Ear cuts occur most frequently to the area between the ear and the head. There will be pain, bleeding, and swelling.

Ear cuts (tears) are caused when the ear is forcefully torn away from the head by a violent twisting action or blow on the ear.

Ear cuts (tears) may be prevented by wearing protective headgear.

Ear cuts (tears) are treated by applying cold to reduce the bleeding. You then must clean the injured area with antiseptic soap and water and apply a sterile pad and wrap. The athlete is taken to the physician for necessary stitches.

Ear cuts (tears) are rehabilitated by keeping the injured area clean and free of infection. Always protect the area with protective padding when the athlete participates.

Foreign Body in Ear

The ear, because of its open structure, is subject to foreign objects becoming lodged in it. There will be discomfort, some pain, and sometimes reduction in hearing.

Foreign bodies in the ear result from flying debris or flying insects.

Foreign bodies in the ear may be prevented by the athlete wearing protective headgear or ear guards in areas where there is a possibility of flying debris or insects.

Foreign bodies in the ear are treated by having the athlete turn his head to one side. If you suspect that the foreign body is an insect, place a light at the ear opening. Usually the insect will crawl out. Should this procedure not work, take a syringe full of luke-warm water and put it in the athlete's ear as he has his head tilted to one side. Let the water stay in the ear for approximately thirty seconds before you have the athlete tilt his ear downward. Be sure you do not strike the ear drum with a direct stream of water. *Never probe for a foreign body in the ear for you might puncture the ear drum.* If after following the above procedure the athlete still complains of discomfort, send him to the physician.

Fungus

Ear fungus is a growth inside the ear and is most common in swimmers. There will be a burning, itching sensation inside the ear.

Ear fungus is caused from excessive moisture inside the ear.

Ear fungus may be prevented by the athlete's wearing ear plugs when in a situation in which the ears are susceptible to moisture.

Ear fungus is treated by washing the inside of the ear with a boric acid and alcohol solution. The best treatment, however, is to send the athlete to a physician to assure that there is nothing more serious than a fungus growth.

EYE INJURIES

The eye is a delicate organ and requires a great deal of care and treatment. You, therefore, must be aware of the symptoms of and the treatments for the following eye injuries. All other injuries in the vicinity of the eye should be treated by the physician.

Burn

Eye burn is not very common but should one occur, you must be able to immediately treat it to prevent permanent damage. In all eye burns there will be impairment of vision, pain, and tears.

Eye burn is caused by a caustic substance coming in contact with the eye.

Eye burn may best be prevented by making sure no caustic substances are used on the field of play or kept in or near the locker facilities.

Eye burn is treated by immediately washing out the eye with clear water, covering with a sterile pad, and sending to the physician. The eye bandage is applied by taking a small gauze pad and placing it over the affected eye. Anchor the patch with an elastic wrap, gauze roll, or cloth around the head.

Eye burn rehabilitation is under the physician's supervision.

Contusion (Black Eye)

An eye contusion is a bruise of the area in and around the eye socket. There will be discoloration, impairment of vision, pain, swelling, and tears.

Eye contusion is caused by a blow to the area of the eye when the athlete is hit or falls against an object.

Eye contusion may be prevented by wearing face masks and eye guards when participating in a sport in which there are flying projectiles.

Eye contusion is immediately treated with cold packs for at least thirty minutes. Be sure to instruct the athlete not to blow his nose for if he does, internal bleeding around the eye will become worse. Next day you may begin heat treatments in the form of moist compresses over the eye. You must be conscious of the temperature of the compresses to prevent blistering the eye area.

Eye contusion rehabilitation consists of the preceding treatment procedures until the eye becomes normal when compared to the athlete's other eye.

Cuts

Eye cuts involve a break in the skin over the eye or a break in the eyeball. The cut over the eye is most common. There will be bleeding, extreme pain, impairment of vision, tears, and a visible opening in the skin or eyeball.

Eye cuts are caused by a sharp point coming into forceful contact with the eye when the athlete is struck by a flying object or another player's fingernail. Cuts over the eye are often caused from a severe blow when the athlete is hit or falls.

Eye cuts may be prevented by making sure the athletes trim their fingernails even with the ends of their fingers, have no sharp edges on their clothing or equipment, and wear face masks.

Eye cuts on the eyeball are covered with a sterile pad and kept in place with a bandage around the head. Then quickly transport the athlete to a physician. Cuts over the eye are treated by lengthwise washing of the wound with antiseptic soap and water, application of an antiseptic, a butterfly patch, and a compression bandage. Then send the athlete to a physician for stitches. You should also apply cold packs to the area to prevent swelling and to stop the bleeding.

Eye cut rehabilitation involves a close watch for infection and daily cleansing and bandaging of the cut. For practice or games provide sufficient protective padding.

Foreign Body in Eye

The eye is immediately disabled by foreign bodies. There will be eye watering, severe pain, and temporary loss of vision.

Foreign bodies in the eye are caused by loose particles flying through the air or by dirt which is blown by the wind into the eye or thrown in the eye when the athlete is tackled or blocked.

Foreign body in the eye because of its nature is rather difficult to prevent.

Foreign body in the eye is treated by irrigating the eye with water or eye wash solution, placing a patch over the eye, and sending the athlete to a physician. However, should you be in a position which requires a length of time before the athlete may reach the physician, you might remove the foreign body from the eye as follows: Hold the upper eye lash between your thumb and forefinger. Then with a cotton-tipped applicator on top of the eye lash, gently turn the eye lash over the cotton-tipped applicator. Have the athlete move his eye up, down, out, and in until you locate the object. When it is located, take another moistened cotton-tipped applicator and gently lift the object from the eye. Then gently lower the eye lash back to its original position. Figure 6-2 illustrates the technique for removing a foreign body from the eye. Be aware that the athlete will experience for a few minutes the sensation of the foreign body's still being in his eye.

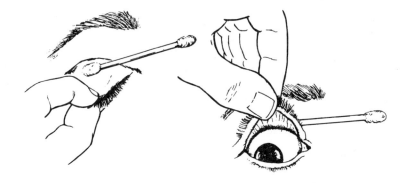

Figure 6-2

FACE INJURIES

Abrasions

Face abrasion is the tearing off of the upper layer or layers of skin resulting in bleeding.

Face abrasion is caused by the athlete's face being scraped against a hard object when he falls, hits another athlete, or is hit by another athlete.

Face abrasion may be prevented by wearing a face mask or other protective gear. Equipment, clothing, and playing areas should be kept free of rough surfaces.

Face abrasion treatment and rehabilitation procedures are the same as those given for abrasion treatment described in Chapter 3.

Burn

Face burn is an inflammation of the skin resulting from friction, heat, or acid.

Face burn is generally caused by overexposure to the sun or by friction.

Face burn may be prevented by applying suntan lotion on the face for prevention of sunburn and skin lubricant on facial areas exposed to friction.

Face burn treatment and rehabilitation procedures are the same as those given for burn treatment in Chapter 3.

Contusion

Face contusion is a bruise on the face area causing superficial damage to the outer layer of skin. It is accompanied by discoloration, pain, and swelling.

Face contusion is caused by a sharp blow to the face when the athlete is hit or falls.

Face contusion may be prevented by wearing protective head gear and face mask.

Face contusion is treated with immediate application of cold for approximately thirty minutes. Next day apply heat to the area.

Face contusion is rehabilitated by frequent application of heat until the injured area is completely free of swelling and discoloration.

Cut

A face cut is the forceful breaking of the skin and surrounding tissue which may be superficial or deep. There will be bleeding, pain, and swelling.

A face cut is caused by a sharp blow to the facial area when the athlete is kicked or bumped by another athlete or when he falls against a sharp object.

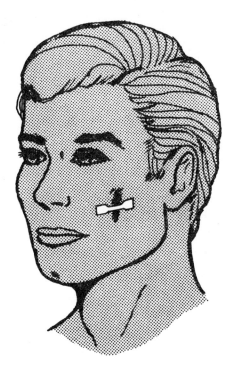

Figure 6-3

A face cut may be prevented with protective equipment, adherence to rules, and elimination of sharp objects from the playing area.

A face cut is treated by lengthwise washing of the wound, applying an antiseptic, and covering with a sterile gauze pad. For the gaping wound, apply a butterfly tape (Figure 6-3) and send the athlete to the physician.

A face cut rehabilitation includes cleanliness of the cut area. You must also keep the area soft so a thick scab will not form. Cover with a sterile gauze pad for practice and games.

Fracture

Face fracture is a breaking or cracking of one of the facial bones. Generally, the face is fractured in the cheekbone area and is sometimes hard to distinguish because of its association with a contused area. There will be discoloration, pain, swelling, and, in extreme cases, a deformity can be noted.

Face fracture is caused by a sharp blow to the face when the athlete is hit by another athlete or when he falls against a hard object.

Face fracture may be prevented by wearing a face mask in those sports in which the face is exposed to hard blows.

Face fracture is treated with cold packs for thirty minutes. Then feel the area with your fingers to detect the break. If the athlete experiences pain when he moves his jaw apply a bandage to immobilize his jaw and transport him to a physician for an X ray to determine the extent of the injury.

MOUTH INJURIES

Cuts

Mouth cuts most often affect the tongue or the lips. Both of these injuries are painful and both will bleed profusely. There will in many instances be swelling.

Mouth cuts are caused by a severe blow to the mouth when the athlete falls or is hit by another athlete. Tongue cuts most often occur when the athlete is hit or falls while he has his tongue between his teeth.

Mouth cuts may be prevented by wearing mouthguards. You might also instruct the athlete to keep his tongue in his mouth when he is actively participating.

Mouth cuts are immediately treated by putting an ice cube in a gauze pad and holding it on the cut until bleeding stops. In gaping wounds, you must take the athlete to a physician for stitches. Be sure to check the tongue and lips to determine whether the cut has completely penetrated the tongue or lip.

Mouth cut rehabilitation involves application of antiseptics and daily washing of the wound. Keep a close watch for infection.

Fractures

Mouth fracture most often involves the teeth and will be very painful. The fracture will be easy to determine since the athlete's teeth will be chipped or completely broken off.

Mouth fracture is caused by a blow to the mouth area or to the chin resulting in the teeth being violently slammed together. This blow may be a result of the athlete's falling or being hit.

Mouth fracture may be prevented by wearing mouthguards and face masks.

Mouth fracture is treated by transporting the athlete to a dentist who will make the necessary corrections.

NOSE INJURIES

Bleeding

Nose bleeding is discharge of blood from one or both nostrils. The bleeding may vary from light to heavy, and the length of bleeding varies from a few minutes to over five minutes. It does not usually disable the athlete but does cause some discomfort or reduction in participation until bleeding is stopped.

Nose bleeding is caused by a direct blow to the nose. It sometimes occurs when the athlete has a jolting fall.

Nose bleeding may be prevented by the athlete's wearing a face mask and mouthguard.

Nose bleeding is treated by applying firm pressure with your thumbs against the upper lip just below the nose (Figure 6-4). Cold compresses just below the nose will also assist in stopping bleeding. Another effective way is to have the athlete seated so that you can comfortably hold his nose. Then gently apply gauze pads in each nostril so that they slightly protrude. Next apply pinching pressure

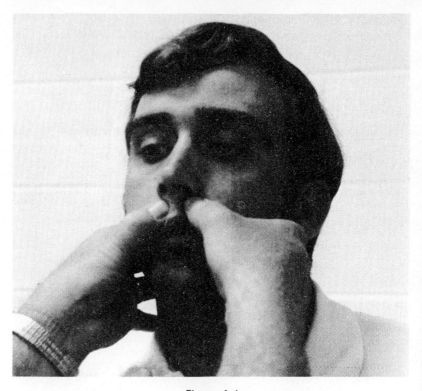

Figure 6-4

with your thumb and forefinger for approximately five to six minutes at which time you gently release the pressure and take out the plugs. If bleeding has not subsided take the athlete to a physician.

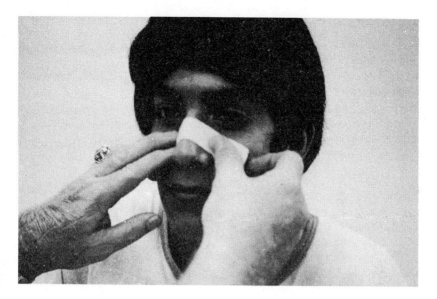

Figure 6-5

Fracture

Nose fracture is a break of the cartilage tissue which forms the nose structure. It will result in bleeding, deformity, discoloration, labored breathing, pain, and tenderness.

Nose fracture is caused by a sharp blow to the nose.

Nose fracture may be prevented by wearing a face mask.

Nose fracture is treated by first stopping the bleeding with cold applications. Then transport the athlete to the physician who will set the nose.

Nose fracture is rehabilitated by applying moist hot compresses to the break. For practice and games, tape the nose as illustrated in Figure 6-5 and be sure to provide a cage guard to prevent further injury. It will take about ten days for the break to heal.

SCALP INJURIES

Cuts

A scalp cut is a break in the skin of the head which will bleed profusely. Generally, there will be pain and swelling and sometimes a headache. Scalp cut is very common in all sports.

Scalp cut is caused by a blow to the head when the athlete is hit or hits an object.

Scalp cut may be prevented by wearing headgear in contact sports.

Scalp cut is treated by applying direct pressure to the bleeding area with a sterile gauze pad wrapped over an ice cube. After bleeding has subsided, cleanse the area with soap and water using a lengthwise motion for cleansing the wound. Apply an antiseptic and a sterile gauze pad. If stitches are needed, take the athlete to a physician.

Scalp cut rehabilitation involves keeping the wound clean and well-protected when the athlete participates.

SKULL INJURY

The skull is composed of eight bones and provides a protective case for the brain. A skull fracture may be present even though there is no visible damage to the scalp. A fracture may occur to any part of the skull, but the most serious is the fracture at the back of the head. An athlete with a skull fracture may have one or all of the following symptoms: unconsciousness, bleeding or oozing of a watery substance from his mouth, nose, or ears, unequal eye pupils which do not respond to light, inability to recall the situation when conscious.

Skull fracture is caused by a violent blow to the head when the athlete is hit or when he falls against a hard object.

Skull fracture may be prevented by wearing protective head gear.

Skull fracture is treated by keeping the athlete on his back so that his head is turned to one side. This will relieve pressure and will keep the athlete from choking should he vomit. It is imperative that you keep the athlete quiet, immobile, warm, and as comfortable as possible. When transporting the athlete to the hospital, you must be certain he is kept on his back on a firm stretcher or board and that he is secured to prevent movement.

7

Neck and Back
Injury Care

The neck and back region is composed of the spinal column which is divided into seven cervical vertebrae, twelve dorsal or thoracic vertebrae, and five lumbar vertebrae. These vertebrae are separated and cushioned by cartilage (discs) and joined by ligaments. These unions provide flexibility at each vertebra so that movement is possible. Because of the spinal column's structure, injuries to it may be very serious, especially if improperly handled. Therefore, you must become familiar with the types of neck and back injuries and their methods of treatment. For you to accomplish this task, neck and back injury care is considered according to the three divisions of the spinal column since injuries to each of these regions will require different handling.

CERVICAL INJURIES (NECK)

Contusion of the Neck

Contusion of the neck is a bruise of the muscles which move the head. There will be pain, swelling, limited motion and sometimes a tingling sensation down the arms. It will usually not disable the athlete, but if it does limit participation, it will only last for one or two days.

Contusion of the neck is caused by a blow to the neck area.

Contusion of the neck may be prevented by adherence to the rules and wearing of protective gear for the shoulder and head in contact sports.

Contusion of the neck is treated by immediate application of cold packs. Next day apply heat and massage to relieve stiffness. If there is excessive stiffness, you might apply a hot pack to the neck area by applying a thin coating of analgesic balm, covering with cotton, and lightly wrapping with an elastic wrap. Be sure the hot pack covers the entire stiff area of the neck. Also, be sure you do not make the wrap too tight.

Contusion of the neck is rehabilitated by adhering to the treatment procedures with the addition of range of motion movements and neck exercises. These exercises are each done for eight seconds.

The exercise for the front neck muscles is administered as follows: Have the athlete lie on his back with his arms palms up at his sides. Place one hand on his chest and the other on his forehead. Then have him try to raise his head against your slight downward pressure (Figure 4-6).

The exercise for the back neck muscles is administered as follows: Have the athlete lie face down with his arms palms up at his sides. Place one hand on his upper back and one hand on the back of his head. Then have him try to raise his head upward and backward against your slight downward pressure (Figure 4-7).

Figures 7-1 and 7-2 show the exercises for the side neck muscles. They are administered as follows: Have the athlete lie on his back or sit with his arms palms up at his sides. Place one hand on the top of his shoulder over the joint and one hand on the side of his head opposite his direction of movement. Then have him try to bring his head to his shoulder.

Contusion of Nerve

Contusion of the neck nerve usually involves the nerve which supplies the arm and hand. It is most often called a pinched nerve and is very painful. There will sometimes be loss of movement accompanied by a tingling sensation in the arm. The numbness sensation resembles the feeling obtained from hitting the "crazy bone" of the elbow. Often there will be a muscle spasm at the point of the injury.

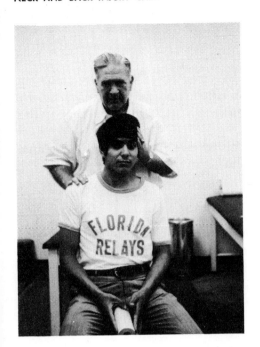

Figure 7-1

Figure 7-2

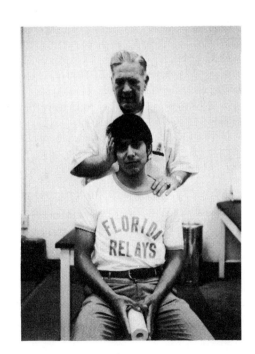

Contusion of the neck nerve is caused by a blow to the neck or a twist which violently snaps the head backward, forward, or sideward.

Contusion of the neck nerve may be prevented by enforcing the face mask holding rule, by eliminating spear tackling, and by wearing protective gear that properly fits. Wearing a neck collar will also help (Figure 4-9).

Contusion of the neck nerve is treated by gently pulling, shaking, and rotating the athlete's arm followed by massage of the arm, neck, and upper shoulder muscles. As soon as you have the sharp pain stopped, you may start applying cold packs to prevent swelling.

Contusion of the neck nerve is rehabilitated by application of heat, massage, and exercises described earlier. You should provide a neck collar when the athlete participates. The procedure for massaging the athlete's neck is fully described in Chapter 4.

Contusion of the Throat

Contusion of the throat usually involves the "Adam's apple." There will be severe pain, coughing with some blood produced, pain when swallowing and talking, and tenderness when the throat area is touched.

Contusion of the throat is caused by a severe blow to the throat area.

Contusion of the throat may be prevented by wearing a neck collar.

Contusion of the throat is immediately treated by applying cold packs to the throat area to prevent internal bleeding. Then take the athlete to the physician so he can check for damage to the air passages. Further treatment and rehabilitation will be under the physician's supervision.

Dislocation

Neck dislocation is a displacement of one or more of the cervical vertebrae from their articular surfaces. There will be severe pain, muscle spasm, a degree of paralysis, and deformity at the back of the neck. There will be a fixed, abnormal position of the head, and any attempt to move the head will result in severe pain.

Neck dislocation is caused by a severe twist or flexion of the neck.

Neck dislocation may be prevented by strengthening the neck and by execution of proper diving and tackling techniques.

Neck dislocation is treated by keeping the athlete quiet and still until a physician or some other competent individual is available for transporting the athlete to a hospital. During transportation, the athlete's neck must be kept stabilized and a rolled up towel should be placed under the curve of his neck. He should also be transported in a backlying position on a firm stretcher.

Neck dislocation rehabilitation begins when the athlete is released by the physician. At this time begin the exercises described earlier in this chapter.

Sprain

Neck sprain occurs when the head is forced beyond its normal range of motion. There will be severe muscle spasms in the neck, shoulder, and upper back region, loss of movement, swelling, and pain on slight movement. In a majority of the cases there will be ligament damage.

Neck sprain is caused by a violent sudden twist, hyperextension, or snap of the head.

Neck sprain may be prevented by strengthening the neck muscles. In football the athlete might prevent the sprain by wearing a neck collar.

Neck sprain is treated by immediate application of cold to reduce swelling. Then have the athlete examined by a physician to rule out neck fracture or dislocation. Next day apply heat, massage, and hot packs to the neck area. Continue until the neck movement returns.

Neck sprain is rehabilitated by continuing heat treatments and exercising the neck muscles with the exercises discussed earlier.

DORSAL SPINE (UPPER BACK)

The dorsal spine (upper back) includes the back area just

below the cervical region to a point approximately one-half way down the spine. It has a very limited range of motion and serves as an attachment for many of the muscles which help move the back. It is subject to contusion, sprain, and strain.

Contusion

A contusion of the upper back region may affect either the muscle or bone or both. It is a common athletic injury but hardly ever disabling. There will be swelling, discoloration, pain, and, in severe cases, muscle spasms.

A contusion of the upper back is caused as a result of the upper back muscles being pressed downward against the spine. This may occur when the athlete is hit or when he falls.

A contusion of the upper back may be prevented with protective padding. Conditioning the muscles of the upper back will help prevent a serious contusion.

A contusion of the upper back is treated by immediately applying cold packs. Next day apply heat and massage.

A contusion of the upper back is rehabilitated by constant application of heat, massage, and by exercises described later in this chapter (see "Exercises" under *Lumbar Spine*).

Sprain

A sprain of the upper back in addition to affecting the muscles usually causes ligament damage. There will be local tenderness on the affected side. Often there will be swelling and dislocation in the injured area because of internal bleeding.

A sprain of the upper back is caused by the back's being violently twisted or hyperextended. Sometimes hyperflexion (bending too far forward) will also result in a dislocation.

A sprain of the upper back may be prevented through strengthening exercises and execution of proper blocking and tackling fundamentals.

A sprain of the upper back is treated with cold packs and immobilization of the athlete until a physician has checked the extent of the injury. Next day start heat treatments.

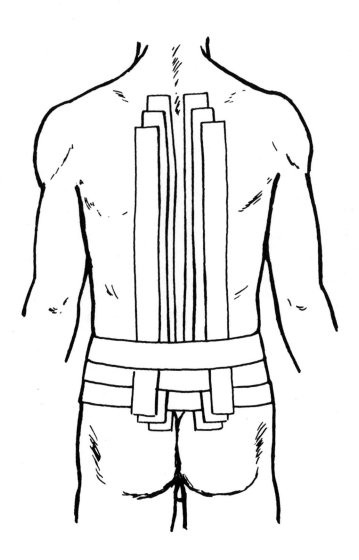

Figure 7-3

A sprain of the upper back is rehabilitated by continuing heat treatments and starting exercises described later (see "Exercises" under *Lumbar Spine*). For practice or games apply tape to prevent excessive movement.

Figure 7-3 illustrates the way to tape an upper back sprain. Prepare the area to be taped by shaving off the body hair and then spraying skin toughener from the base of the neck to the top of the buttocks. Using three-inch tape apply a vertical strip of tape on each side of the spine. Next put a horizontal strip of tape across the top of the buttocks so that it goes around each of the athlete's sides. After this alternately place vertical strips in an overlapping manner on each side of the spine until you have covered approximately three-fourths of the athlete's back. Anchor the ends of the vertical strips by placing horizontal strips just below the neck and just above the buttocks.

Strain

A strain of the upper back involves several or all of the muscles in this area. There will be spasms, severe pain, and swelling. Movement will be painful, and the athlete will experience stiffness in the upper back.

A strain of the upper back is caused when the upper back muscles are jerked or twisted past their normal range of movement. There will be severe pain, localized tenderness, and some swelling.

A strain of the upper back may be prevented by strengthening the muscles.

A strain of the upper back is immediately treated with cold applications. Next day apply heat and light massage. If a spasm is still present, ask the physician for muscle relaxants. Give these muscle relaxants only as prescribed by the physician.

A strain of the upper back is rehabilitated by heat treatments and the exercises described below (under *Lumbar Spine*). For practice or games tape the athlete's back to prevent excessive movement. The correct taping method has been described (Figure 7-3).

LUMBAR SPINE (LOWER BACK)

The lower back region includes the area between the pelvic

girdle and the chest cavity. Unlike the upper back, it is very movable and stable. Common injuries with which you should be familiar are contusions and sprains.

Contusion

A contusion of the lower back generally involves the muscles, even though the bone may sometimes be affected. This is not a severe injury and will cause no loss of practice or game time. There will, however, be pain and localized tenderness.

A contusion of the lower back is caused by a blow to the area.

A contusion of the lower back may be prevented with protective padding.

A contusion of the lower back is immediately treated with cold applications to reduce swelling. Next day apply heat and light stretching.

A contusion of the lower back is rehabilitated by application of heat, massage, hot packs, and the exercises described later. The hot pack is applied by placing a thin coating of analgesic balm on the back, covering with cotton, and wrapping with an elastic wrap.

Sprain

A sprain of the lower back involves the muscles and ligaments. There will be pain on movement, stiffness, loss of movement, localized tenderness, and swelling.

A sprain of the lower back is caused when the lower back is severely twisted or bent past its normal range of motion.

A sprain of the lower back may be prevented by strengthening the low back muscles.

A sprain of the lower back is treated with immediate application of cold packs and a compression bandage. Next day apply heat, stretching exercises, and a hot pack like that described above.

A sprain of the lower back is rehabilitated by constant adherence to treatment procedures and the addition of the exercises described later. For practice and games apply tape to the low back region as described below and illustrated in Figure 7-4. First prepare the area to be taped by shaving off the body hair and spraying with skin toughener. Apply horizontal strips of tape starting just above the buttocks and continuing until the tape reaches just above the top of the pelvis. These strips of tape anchor near the front of the athlete's body. Next apply strips of tape at an angle so that they form an "X" near the center of the taped area. Then apply vertical anchor strips on the ends of the tape on the front of the athlete's body.

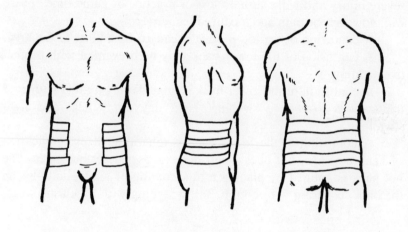

Figure 7-4

Exercises

Isometric   The following isometric exercises are performed twice daily for eight seconds.

Figure 7-5 illustrates the exercise for the upper back. It is administered as follows: Have the athlete lie face down on a table with his hands clasped behind his head. Place your hand on his upper shoulders, and with your other hand hold his hips down. Then have him raise his upper body against your downward pressure.

Figure 7-6 illustrates an exercise for the lower back. It is administered as follows: Have the athlete lie on his stomach with his arms palms up at his sides. Grasp his lower leg at the ankle. Then have the athlete try to raise his leg upward without bending it

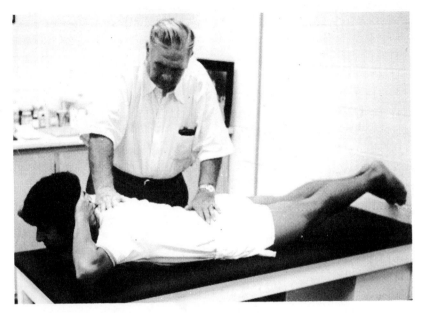

Figure 7-5

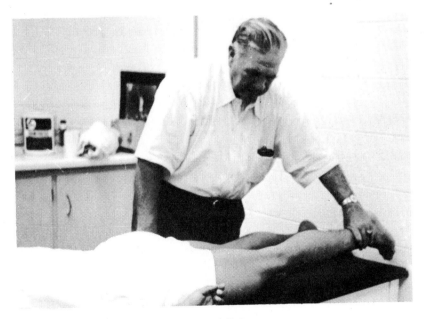

Figure 7-6

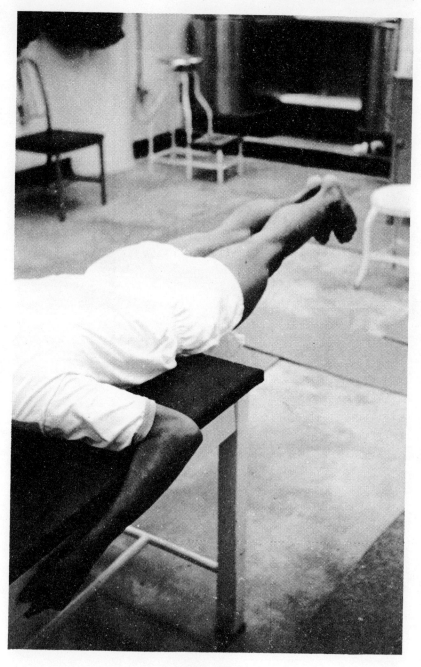

Figure 7-7

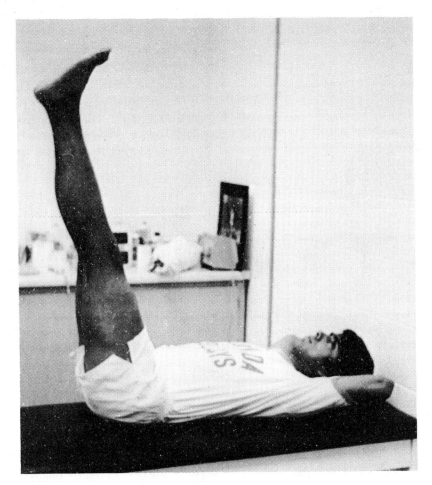

Figure 7-8

as you apply downward pressure. Alternate legs to assure both areas of the lower back are being strengthened.

Isotonic   The following isotonic exercises may be performed with or without weights. When you use weights follow the procedure outlined in Chapter 5.

Figure 7-7 illustrates the reverse leg raise. It is administered as follows: Have the athlete lie face down on a table so that his hips are supported by the end of the table and his legs hang downward. Have him grasp the edge of the table and while keeping his

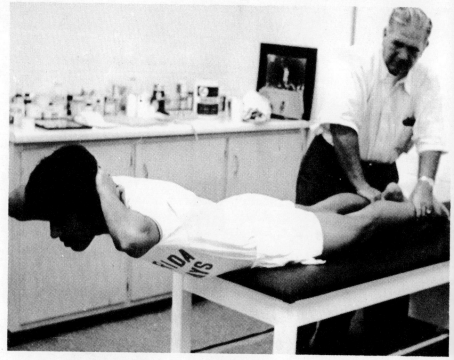

Figure 7-9

legs straight raise them as high as possible before returning them to the starting position.

Figure 7-8 illustrates the regular leg lift. It is administered as follows: Have the athlete lie on his back so that his legs are straight. Then have him raise his legs as high as possible without bending the knees.

Figure 7-9 illustrates the trunk raise. It is administered as follows: Have the athlete lie face down on a table so that his upper body hangs over the end of the table. Then anchor his legs by holding them or strapping them to the table. Next have him clasp his hands behind his neck and alternately raise and lower his upper body as far in each direction as he can go.

8

Trunk Injury Care

The trunk of the body is the area between the base of the neck and the bottom of the pelvis. It encloses the vital organs, supports the neck and head, and provides an attachment for the arms and legs. It is divided into the abdominal cavity, which includes the area from the diaphragm down through the pelvis, and the chest cavity, which includes the area up from the diaphragm to the base of the neck. Trunk injuries include kidney, muscle, rib, spleen, sternum, stitch-in-side, testes, and wind-knocked-out.

KIDNEY INJURY

The kidneys are located in the lower part of the back near the bottom of the ribs. Kidney injuries will vary from moderate (contusion) to severe (rupture). In the moderate (contused), there will be some blood in the urine as well as mild pain extending over a few days. In a severe (ruptured) kidney injury, there will be sharp, intense pain in the back, swelling, blood in the urine, muscle spasms in the back, shock, nausea, and vomiting.

Kidney injury is caused by a sharp blow to the lower back or abdominal region.

Kidney injury may be prevented by having the athlete wear protective pads.

Kidney injury treatment is under the direct supervision of the physician. However, until you are absolutely sure, or until the physician arrives, you should apply cold packs to the area which was hit. Be sure to keep the athlete quiet. Never let the athlete return to competition until you are convinced he has no real kidney damage.

MUSCLE INJURY

The trunk muscles include the abdominal, back, and chest muscles. These muscles like all muscles are subject to bruises, contusions, and strains. Refer to Chapter 5 for the correct procedures for treating bruises, contusions, and strains.

RIB INJURY

The ribs form the outer wall for the chest cavity and protect the heart and lungs. They are most often subject to dislocations (or separations) or fractures.

Dislocation

Rib dislocation involves one or more of the ribs being forced out of its jointure with the cartilage tissue located between the rib cage and the sternum (breast bone). There will be sharp pain on movement of the chest wall, and, in many cases, there is a deformity on the athlete's chest.

Rib dislocation is caused by a sharp blow, twisting, or stretching of the rib cage.

Rib dislocation may be prevented with protective padding and by strengthening the abdominal, back, and chest muscles.

Rib dislocation treatment includes use of cold packs and pressure for reducing swelling and deformity. Never attempt to reduce a rib dislocation except in cases of extreme emergency. If you must reduce the deformity, have the athlete lie on his back, take a deep breath, and hold it as another person moves his shoulder backward. At the same time, you apply firm pressure with the heel of your hand to force the rib back into position. Be sure you do not apply too much pressure or you may puncture the lung. After you

have the rib in place, cover the dislocated area with a felt pad and
tape it into position with three inch tape. Figure 8-1 illustrates the
technique for taping the ribs. Have the athlete either sitting or
standing with his arm raised over the affected side. Cover the
breast with a gauze pad and spray the chest and back area with skin
toughener. Next place a vertical strip of tape approximately seven
or eight inches long down the center of the athlete's chest and back.
Bring a horizontal strip of tape from the bottom of the vertical strip
in the back around to the bottom of the vertical strip on the front.
Continue this procedure so that the tape overlaps the previous strip
approximately half way. Follow this pattern until you have covered
the area all the way to the top of the vertical strip.

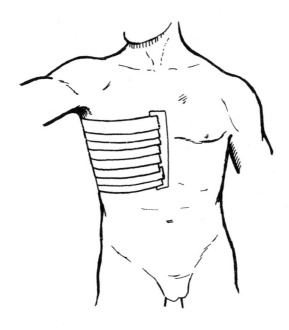

Figure 8-1

Rib dislocation rehabilitation proceeds under the close supervision of the physician. At this time, you start heat treatment and
hot packs and continue for approximately three to six weeks.

Fracture

Rib fracture occurs frequently in contact sports and may involve one or more of the ribs. There will be a sharp localized pain
when the athlete takes a deep breath, coughs, or sneezes, or when
you apply pressure to his rib cage. The athlete also tends to carry
his head forward and breathe easily to lessen pain. In extreme cases
the athlete may cough up blood.

Rib fracture is caused by a sharp, direct blow to the rib cage.
It may also be caused by a violent twist, stretch, or pressure on the
rib cage.

Rib fracture may be prevented by the athlete's wearing protective padding and participating in strength programs.

Rib fracture treatment consists of first making a correct
assessment of the injury. In all cases of severe blows to the chest
area where there is sharp pain on normal movement, be sure to
have the athlete's chest X-rayed. Until you get the athlete to a
physician for the X ray, apply cold packs to reduce swelling. When
the athlete is coughing up blood, place him on a stretcher with his
head elevated and quickly transport him to a hospital. During this
stage, you must make certain the athlete is not jolted.

Rib fracture rehabilitation is directly supervised by the
physician. For practice and games the athlete's ribs are taped as
illustrated in Figure 8-1.

SPLEEN

Spleen injuries are complicated and frequently appear not
serious. Then the athlete may suddenly die after a period of hours,
days, or weeks. Therefore, anytime an athlete is hit in the abdominal area, watch for mild shock, tenderness in the upper left corner
of the abdomen toward the back, and localized pain. When the
spleen is severely damaged, the athlete will experience pain in the

left shoulder and approximately a third of the way down the left arm.

Spleen injuries are caused by the athlete's falling, being blocked, or being crushed.

Spleen injuries may be prevented by the athlete's use of protective trunk pads and execution of proper blocking fundamentals.

Spleen injury treatment involves specific questioning of the athlete who has suffered a blow to the abdominal region. At the same time, you must check for rigid abdominal muscles, signs of shock, nausea, vomiting, or pain in the left shoulder and arm (Kehr's Sign). When you suspect any of these conditions, quickly transport the athlete to a physician or a hospital.

STERNUM INJURIES

The sternum (breast bone) is the flat bone in the center of the chest. It provides an attachment for the rib cartilage and is subject to contusions and fractures.

Contusions

Sternum contusion is damage to the bone covering. There will be pain, swelling, tenderness, and sometimes a deformity.

Sternum contusion is caused by a sharp blow to the breast bone.

Sternum contusion may be prevented by the athlete's wearing protective pads on the chest area.

Sternum contusion is immediately treated with cold. Next day apply heat and hot packs. When a deformity is present, take the athlete to the physician for treatment.

Fracture

Sternum fracture results in pain at point of fracture when the athlete is breathing. There will be swelling, possible deformity, and pain when the athlete holds his head in a normal position. There will also be tenderness when you feel the injured area.

Sternum fracture is caused by a sharp blow to the upper chest area.

Sternum fracture may be prevented by the athlete's wearing protective padding for the chest area.

Sternum fracture is treated by a physician. You must transport the athlete in a backlying position on a firm stretcher. Be cautious during the transporting to prevent the broken bones from causing excessive damage to the surrounding tissue.

STITCH-IN-SIDE

Stitch-in-the-side is the term used for the rapid, severe pain which affects either the left or right side of many athletes, especially basketball and track participants.

Stitch-in-the-side's cause is not known, but it is thought the condition may be a result of the athlete's being constipated, having gas in his stomach, eating too fast, or fatiguing the diaphragm.

Stitch-in-the-side may be prevented by moderate eating on the part of the athlete and through progressive conditioning programs which emphasize strengthening the abdominal muscles.

Stitch-in-the-side is treated by raising the athlete's arm above his head in order to stretch the affected side. You may also gently rub the affected area.

TESTES

The testes are susceptible to injury because of their exposed position. There will be immediate, severe pain, faintness, and sometimes swelling.

Testes injuries occur when the athlete is sharply hit by a blow from a helmet, fist, or foot.

Testes injuries may be prevented by the athlete's wearing a plastic guard (cup) in his supporter when he engages in a contact sport.

Testes injuries are immediately treated with the following method: Have the athlete lie on his back. Then gently bend his knees to his chest until the pain subsides. You may, if feasible, apply cold packs to prevent swelling.

If the athlete still complains of pain after you have treated him, take him to the training room and examine his scrotum for swelling or testicular displacement. If either of these conditions is present, have a physician examine the athlete.

WIND-KNOCKED-OUT

Wind-knocked-out involves the momentary stoppage of the breathing processes. The athlete cannot breathe and will feel faint, nauseous, and weak.

Wind-knocked-out is caused by the athlete's being unexpectedly hit in the abdominal region when these muscles are relaxed.

Wind-knocked-out is best prevented by the athlete's always having the abdominal muscles tensed during all phases of competition.

Wind-knocked-out is treated by asking the athlete to inhale slowly through his nose and exhale through his mouth. While he is doing this, you should be loosening clothing or equipment around the neck and chest area so he has more freedom to breathe. Another good procedure is to have the athlete lie on his back and bend his knees so his thighs touch his chest. *Never lift the athlete by his belt.* Be sure you check for all the symptoms of internal organ damage.

9

Leg Injury Care

The leg is divided into the upper and lower legs. Its primary purpose is to furnish support and locomotion for the athlete.

UPPER LEG

The upper leg is composed of the femur (thigh bone), quadriceps (front thigh muscle), and hamstrings (back thigh muscles). Injuries which affect the upper leg are muscle contusion, bone fracture, and muscle strains.

Contusion

Contusion of the upper leg is commonly referred to as a charley horse. Its nature, cause, prevention, and treatment has been fully described in Chapter 5. However, its taping procedure has not been previously explained. Figure 9-1 shows the method for taping an upper leg contusion. Prepare the area to be taped by shaving off the hair and spraying with skin toughener. Have the athlete stand with his heel elevated approximately one-and-a-half inches. Start at a point about four inches above the kneecap by applying a horizontal strip of tape half way around the athlete's leg. Continue this taping procedure, overlapping the bottom strip half-way until you have completely covered the upper leg. Next apply diagonal strips of tape from the left bottom corner to the right upper corner and then apply another diagonal strip in the opposite way.

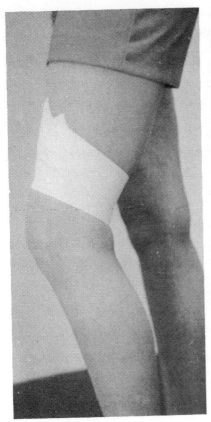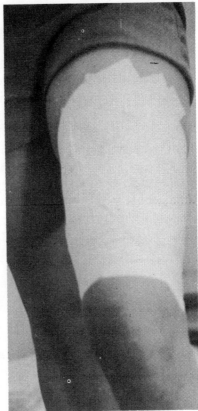

Figure 9-1

Continue until you have covered the entire thigh area. After completing the taping job cover the entire area with an elastic wrap.

Fracture

Fracture of the upper leg involves the shaft of the femur. There will be deformity, muscle spasms, pain, tenderness, swelling, loss of motion, shortening of the thigh, and the affected foot will be turned outward.

Fractures are caused by a sharp blow or kick to the upper leg or a pileup on the leg. Sometimes the athlete's upper leg may be broken when he jumps or falls from a great height.

Fracture may be prevented by strengthening the thigh muscles, enforcing the piling on rules, and providing soft, absorbent material for the athlete to land on when he must fall from great heights.

Fractures are treated by applying a splint and transporting the athlete to a physician or hospital. Immobilize the upper leg fracture by placing one splint on the outside of the leg from under the arm down the outside of the leg to the ankle and one splint on the inside of the leg from the groin down to the ankle. Then anchor it with tape or bandages at the ankle, just below the knee, just above the knee, and just below the groin. If you have no splinting materials available, tie both the athlete's legs together and transport him on a stretcher. It is important that you prevent the onset of shock by keeping the athlete warm and comfortable.

Strain

Strain in the upper leg usually affects the hamstring muscles. There will be severe pain, swelling, discoloration, and loss of movement.

Strain of the upper leg is caused by unequal muscle development, fatigue, lack of salt in the diet, improper warmup exercises, lack of condition, sudden temperature change, or a sudden jerk on the muscle from a change in direction.

Strain of the upper leg may be prevented by strengthening and stretching exercises, increased salt in the athlete's diet, proper warmups, and prevention of fatigue.

Strains of the upper leg are immediately treated with cold applications and a compression wrap from the knee up to the buttocks. Next day apply heat, massage, and hot packs.

Strains of the upper leg are rehabilitated by applying heat, massage, hot pack, and exercises.

Figure 9-2 illustrates the *isometric* exercise for the lower hamstring muscle. It is administered as follows: Have the athlete lie on his stomach on a table with his arms palms up at his sides. Place your hand on his heel and have him raise his leg high enough for you to place your fist thumb side up under his leg. While his leg is in this position, apply gentle pressure while he tries to raise his leg.

Figure 9-3 illustrates the isometric exercise for the middle

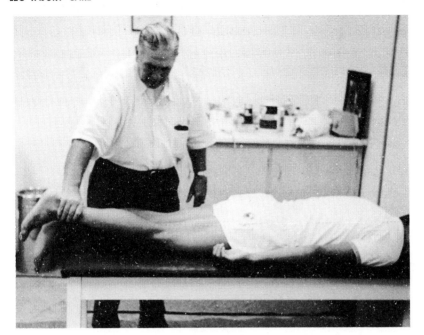

Figure 9-2

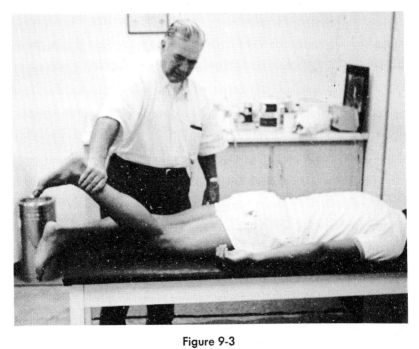

Figure 9-3

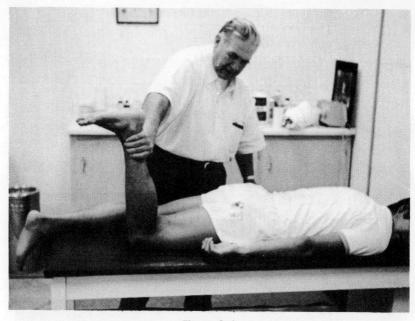

Figure 9-4

hamstring muscle. It is administered with the athlete in the same position described in Figure 9-2. The difference is that the athlete brings his lower leg to a 45-degree angle. You then apply gentle pressure on his heel as he tries to bring his heel to his back.

Figure 9-4 illustrates the isometric exercise for the upper hamstring. It is administered with the athlete in the same position described in Figure 9-2. This exercise requires the athlete to bring his lower leg up so it forms a 90-degree angle with his body. Apply pressure on his heel as he attempts to move it toward his back.

An *isotonic* exercise for the hamstring strain is administered according to the procedure outlined in Chapter 5. With the athlete lying on his stomach, attach the weight to his heel and have him move his lower leg through a full range of motion.

LOWER LEG

The lower leg is composed of the tibia (large bone or shin bone) and the fibula (small bone) as well as the calf and front leg muscles. The bones of the leg are subject to fracture and the muscles are subject to contusion, shin splints, and strain.

Contusion

Contusion of the lower leg affects the calf muscles or the shins. There will be pain, loss of movement, swelling, discoloration, and, in the case of the calf muscles, muscle spasms.

Contusion of the lower leg is caused by a sharp blow when the athlete is hit or kicked or bumps into an object.

Contusion of the lower leg is difficult to prevent due to the lower leg's exposed position. However, in contact sports, the athlete may wear shin protectors.

Contusion of the lower leg is immediately treated with cold packs, compression bandages, and elevation of the leg. Next day apply heat, massage, and hot packs.

Contusion of the lower leg is rehabilitated with heat treatments and exercises for the calf muscles. These exercises consist of the athlete's rising on his toes with his knees straight and then with his knees bent. To stretch the injured area, the athlete should stand facing a wall at arm's length and then lean forward without lifting his heels from the floor. He can also stretch the calf muscles by standing on a step so his heels are hanging over the edge. Then he lowers his heels as far as possible.

Hot pack   Hot pack for the lower leg is applied by spreading a thin coating of analgesic balm over the bruised area, covering with cotton, and wrapping from the ankle to the knee with an elastic wrap.

Fracture

Fracture of the lower leg most often affects the fibula. Fibula fractures are sometimes not immediately noticeable since it is not a weight-bearing bone. Conversely a fracture of the tibia will be immediately noticeable since the athlete will experience pain when walking or will not be able to walk. Fractures of either lower leg bone will cause pain, loss of movement, deformity, swelling, and sometimes bleeding or shock.

Fracture of the lower leg is caused when the athlete suffers a sharp blow or bending of the lower leg bone.

Fracture of the lower leg is best prevented by enforcing rules of play and by strengthening the athlete's lower leg muscles.

Fracture of the lower leg is treated by a physician. To transport the athlete to the physician, apply a splint on each side of the leg from the knee down below the ankle. Anchor it in place with tape or cloth bandages.

Shin Splints

Shin splints affect the lower front of the shin. There will be pain in the lower leg when the athlete puts weight on his foot, the shin will be tender to the touch, and you will feel rough sandlike protrusions under the skin when you run your fingers along the shin bone.

Shin splint cause is not known, but is thought to be a result of dropped arches, pulled muscles, the athlete's running on his toes before he is in shape, inflammation, muscle spasms, strained muscles, or the athlete's running on hard surfaces.

Shin splints may be prevented by properly conditioning the athlete before he runs on a hard surface, immediately treating any soreness in the shin area, applying tape under the arches, and strengthening the lower leg muscles.

Shin splints are treated with rest and heat. If the athlete must play, he should also heat the shin area for approximately 20 or 30 minutes. Never let him play if he cannot walk without sharp pain.

Shin splints are rehabilitated with constant heat on the shin area along with exercise for strength and tape for support.

An exercise for the front leg muscles is administered as follows: Have the athlete sit on a table with his lower leg, toes pointed downward, extending about six inches over the edge of the table. Place your hand on his toes and one on the bottom of his heel. Then have him try to bring his toe toward his body as you apply resistance.

Figure 9-5 illustrates the tape technique for shin splints. It is administered as follows: Prepare the shin and foot by shaving off the hair and spraying with skin toughener. Apply horizontal strips

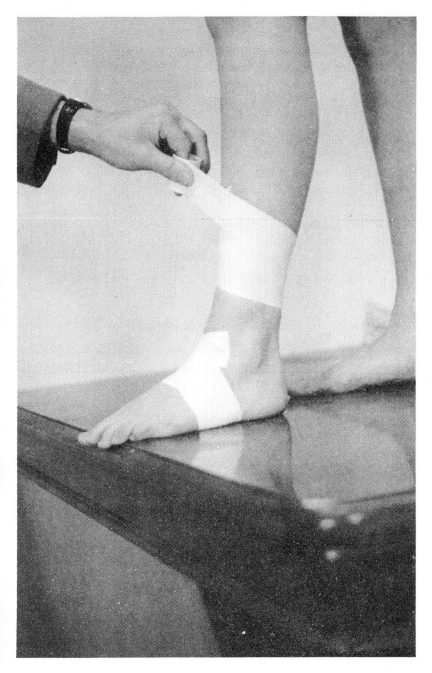

Figure 9-5

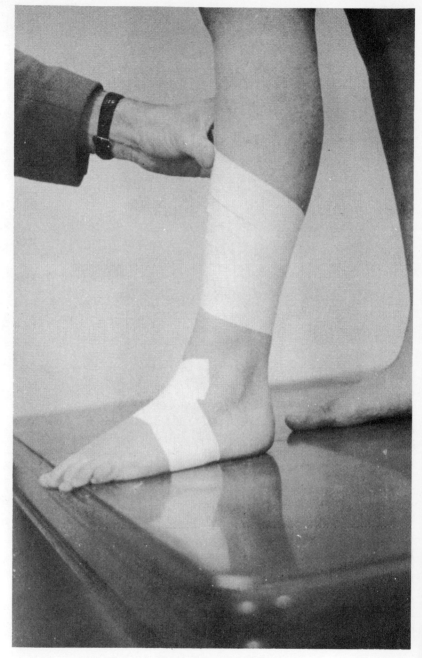

Figure 9-5 continued

around the arch of the foot with a slight lifting motion. Then starting just above the ankle bone, apply horizontal strips of tape, so that they overlap about half way, up to the base of the calf muscle. Be sure you pull the tape toward the front of the leg where it is attached. This is the tape technique I found most effective. You may have to experiment since all shin splints differ.

Strain

Strain of the lower leg generally affects the calf muscle. There will be pain, loss of movement, tightness, swelling, and sometimes discoloration.

Strain of the lower leg is caused by the muscle's being forced beyond its normal range of motion when it is not properly warmed before exertion.

Strain of the lower leg may be prevented by strengthening and stretching exercises for the lower leg and adequate warmup before the athlete participates. Also, when the athlete feels a tightness in the calf of his muscle, he must not try to walk it out.

Strain of the lower leg is immediately treated with cold packs and compression bandages, rest, and elevation of the leg as much as possible. Next day apply heat, massage, and hot packs.

Strain of the lower leg is rehabilitated with rest, heat, massage, hot pack, stretching, and exercise.

An isometric exercise for the calf muscles is administered as follows: Have the athlete sit on a table so that his foot is at a 90-degree angle with his leg and extended about six inches over the edge of the table. Place one of your hands behind his heel, and with your other hand hold the bottom of his foot just below his toes as he tries to push his foot away from his body.

10

Foot Injury Care

The foot has three divisions consisting of the back part made up of the calcaneus (heel bone) and talus; the center part which includes the navicular, cuboid, and cuniforms; and the front part made up of the metatarsals and phalanges (toes).

The primary function of the foot is to transmit the weight of the body down through the leg to the surface and to provide flexibility for locomotion.

EXAMINATION

When the athlete experiences foot trouble, you must closely examine his foot for external blemishes or deformity, compare the injured foot with the uninjured foot, and gently feel and manipulate the heel area, the bottom and top of the foot, and the toes.

TREATMENT

The above examination of the foot will usually identify one or more of the following foot disorders: athlete's foot, blister, bunion, bursitis, callus, corn, contusion, dislocation, fracture, hammer toe, ingrown toenail, plantar wart, sprain, strain or tenosynovitis.

Athlete's Foot

A complete description of and the treatment procedure for athlete's foot is contained in Chapter 4.

Blister

A complete description of and the treatment procedure for blisters is contained in Chapter 4.

Bunion

A complete description of and the treatment procedure for bunions is contained in Chapter 4.

Bursitis

Bursitis of the foot is an inflammation of either of the bursa located between the heel bone and the skin on the underside of the foot or the bursa between the achilles tendon and the heel bone. There will be pain when you press either of these affected areas or when the athlete puts pressure on either of the bursa.

Bursitis of the foot is caused by a constant irritation on the heel area from poorly fitted shoes, hard surfaces, bumping of the heel, or inattention to bruises.

Bursitis of the foot may be prevented by immediately treating any bruise to the heel area, wearing sponge rubber or a heel cup on the heel, and by properly fitting the athlete's shoes.

Bursitis of the foot is treated with heat treatments and protective pads. The physician might also locally inject the bursae.

Bursitis of the foot rehabilitation involves constant use of heat and sponge rubber pads in the athlete's shoes. Be certain you eliminate all possible sources of severe pressure on the heel area.

Callus

A complete description of and the treatment procedure for calluses is contained in Chapter 4.

Corn

A complete description of and the treatment procedure for corns is contained in Chapter 4.

Contusion

Contusion of the foot is common in athletics and sometimes develops into serious problems because of inattention. Generally, contusions occur on the bottom surface of the foot at the heel or ball of the foot. However, contusions may also occur on the top or side of the foot. There will be pain when weight or pressure is applied to the foot, swelling, discoloration, slight loss of movement, and, in extreme cases, nerve damage.

Contusion of the foot is caused by the athlete's being hit by another athlete, dropping something on his foot, or stepping hard on a sharp protusion. Faulty cleats, wrinkled socks, or broken soles on the shoes also contribute to foot contusion.

Contusion of the foot may be prevented by providing the athlete with good shoes and fitted socks, sponge pads in shoes, wearing a heel cup, and elimination of sharp objects from the playing surface.

Contusion of the foot is immediately treated with cold packs and distribution of the weight so it does not place stress on the contused area of the foot. Next day apply heat, and place sponge rubber in the shoe or on the bottom of the foot to distribute the weight off the contused area. Continue these treatments until the athlete experiences no pain when pressure is applied to the foot.

Contusion on the heel area is more handicapping than other foot contusions, and it must be frequently treated with heat. When the athlete participates, you must protect the heel from further bruising by providing the athlete with a heel cup or a felt or sponge rubber pad. For very painful heel contusion, you will have to provide tape to prevent pressure. Figure 10-1 illustrates the method for taping the heel contusion. Have the athlete sit on a table with his foot extended over the edge of the table. Stand in front of him and apply a one-and-one-half inch tape around the back of the heel to a point just in front of and below the ankle protrusions. Next apply a strip of tape under the heel near the back of the athlete's ankle up to the previous horizontal strip. Alternate this pattern until you have completely enclosed the heel area. Be sure to apply quite a bit of pressure to assure firm support.

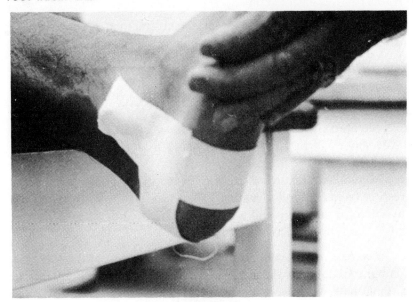

Figure 10-1

Dislocation

Dislocation in the foot area most often concerns the toes. There will be an obvious deformity, pain, swelling, and eventually discoloration.

Dislocation of the toe is caused when the toe is forced from its normal jointure by a blow to the side or front of the toe.

Dislocation of the toe may be prevented by the athlete's wearing sturdy-toed shoes.

Dislocation of the toe is treated by transporting the athlete to the physician. Never try to reduce the dislocation.

Dislocation of the toe rehabilitation starts after about two weeks. It consists of heat, massage, and exercises. Continue this procedure until the athlete can walk without pain. The exercise for the toes consist of the athlete's using his toes to pick up a pencil, towel, or marbles from the floor.

Fracture

Fracture of the foot most commonly involves the second or third metatarsals and the toes.

Metatarsal Fracture   Metatarsal fracture involves either the second or third metatarsal just behind the second or third toe. There will be pain, swelling, some deformity, and inability to support the weight of the body without a limp.

Metatarsal fracture is caused by a direct, violent force to the athlete's foot or by fatigue (March Fracture).

Metatarsal fracture may be prevented by the athlete's wearing sturdy shoes and by elimination of heavy exercise when the athlete is fatigued.

Metatarsal fracture is treated by applying cold packs, compression bandage, and elevation. Then transport the athlete to the physician for an X ray and a cast. All other treatment procedure is under direct supervision of the physician.

Toe Fracture   Toe fracture may affect any of the toes, but it is most frequent in the big toe. Symptoms include discoloration, swelling, pain when weight must be borne, and tenderness over the point of the break.

Toe fracture is caused by a direct, violent blow on the toes either from the athlete's being stepped on, hitting his toes against something, or by his dropping a heavy object on his toes.

Toe fracture may be prevented by having the athlete wear sturdy shoes with stiff toe areas. He should never be allowed to participate in a contact sport without shoes.

Toe fracture is immediately treated with cold to reduce swelling. After about 20 minutes, place a felt pad between the fractured toe and its adjacent toe and tape them together, apply more ice as you are transporting the athlete to the physician. All other treatment will be under the direct supervision of the physician.

Hammer Toe

Hammer toe is a condition in which the athlete's toes are forced into a claw-like position (Figure 10-2). There will be a definite deformity and discomfort when the athlete walks.

Hammer toe develops when the athlete wears shoes which are too short.

Hammer toe may be prevented by making sure the athlete's shoes properly fit in the toe area.

Hammer toe is treated by soaking the foot in a hot water bath

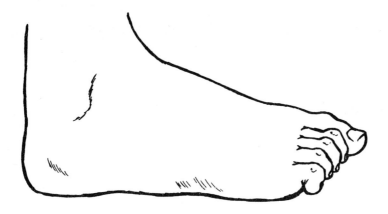

Figure 10-2

and then forcing the toes straight. Next cut from felt material a toe pad according to the pattern in Figure 10-3. Make sure you put the beveled edge under the big toe.

Hammer toe rehabilitation simply involves constant continuation of the treatment procedure.

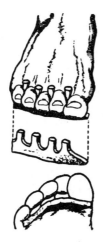

Figure 10-3

Ingrown Toenail

A complete description of and the treatment procedure for ingrown toenail is contained in Chapter 4.

Plantar Wart

A complete description of and the treatment procedure for a plantar wart is contained in Chapter 4.

Sprain

Foot sprains affect the longitudinal arch, the toes, or the transverse arch.

Longitudinal Arch   The longitudinal arch runs from the heel to the back of the toes and is considered to be the main arch in the foot. When it is sprained, it will tend to drop, causing pain in the middle of the foot on the bottom side due to stretched or torn ligaments. There will be sharp pain on walking, and sometimes walking may be impossible.

Longitudinal arch sprain is caused by the bones and ligaments of the arch being forced beyond their normal range when the athlete places a violent stress on his foot.

Longitudinal arch sprains may be prevented by strengthening the muscles of the lower leg and by not forcing the athlete into a situation where he must place excessive stress on his feet when he is tired. You may also apply tape around the arch or place a felt pad under the arch when the athlete first experiences pain.

Longitudinal arch sprain is treated with cold packs and compression bandage around his arch. Next day apply heat.

Longitudinal arch sprain is rehabilitated by frequent applications of heat. After heat treatments, apply tape for support. Figure 10-4 shows how to tape the arch. Spray the bottom of the foot with skin toughener. Apply an anchor strip of one-inch tape across the bottom of the foot at the base of the toes. Then starting at the big toe joint take the tape alongside the bottom of the foot, around the heel, and back to the big toe joint. Start the next strip of tape under the little toe joint, go alongside the bottom of the foot, around the

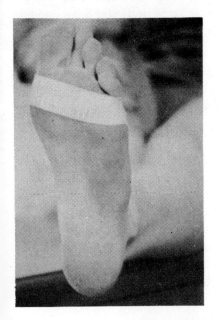
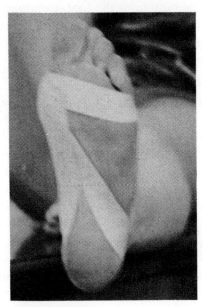
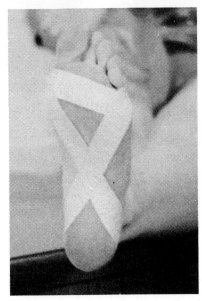

Figure 10-4

heel, and back to the little toe joint. The tape now forms an "X" on
the bottom of the foot. Continue these steps until you have enough
tape to support the athlete's arch so that he can move without
difficulty.

     Toe Sprain   Sprains in the toe area result when the toe is
forced beyond its normal range of motion. There will be a slight
deformity, pain, tenderness, and swelling. When the big toe is
sprained, the athlete will be unable to rise on his toes. He will also
experience pain when he walks.

     Toe sprains are caused when the athlete stubs his toe or twists
it past its normal range of movement.

     Toe sprains may be prevented by the athlete's wearing shoes
in contact sports or by taping the toes together in sports when shoes
cannot be worn or when the athlete has a weak toe.

     Toe sprains are treated by soaking the toes in a cold water
bath for approximately 30 to 45 minutes. Then immobilize the
joint by taping a three-eighths inch felt pad on the athlete's foot
(Figure 10-5). Next day apply heat.

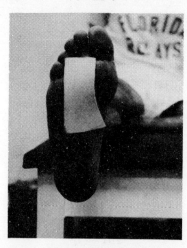

Figure 10-5

     Toe sprains are rehabilitated by frequent heat treatments,
application of the foot pad, and taping a small block of wood or
metal under the athlete's street shoe just behind his big toe. Tape
the athlete's toe whenever he participates. When a small toe is involved, tape it to the adjacent good toe to alleviate pain. Big toe
sprain taping is illustrated in Figure 10-6. Start a strip of one-inch
tape on the side of the foot at the jointure of the big toe with the

foot, go between the big toe and the next toe, around the big toe, across the foot, and under the foot back to the starting place.

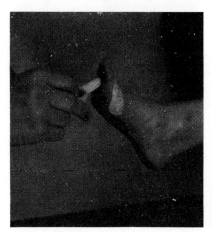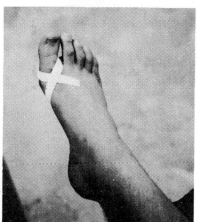

Figure 10-6

Transverse Arch Sprain   Transverse arch sprain affects the area under the ball of the foot. The athlete will first experience redness and irritation on the ball of the foot and pain when he applies pressure to this area. If the condition is not quickly corrected, there will be toe cramping, callus formation, and sometimes a burning sensation.

Transverse arch sprain is caused by a prolonged stress on the athlete's feet from moving or standing on a hard surface.

Transverse arch sprain may be prevented by application of a metatarsal pad as soon as the athlete feels pain in the ball of the foot.

Transverse arch sprain is treated with heat, massage, exercise, and metatarsal pads. Figure 10-7 shows how to apply the metatarsal pad. Have the athlete sit or lie on a table so that his foot forms a right angle with his leg. Place a two inch circular felt pad just behind the second, third, and fourth toes. Then with one-and-a-half inch tape, secure the pad.

Transverse arch sprain exercises include (a) pushing the foot downward; (b) lifting the toes upward; (c) bending the toes; (d) grasping a towel with the toes; and (e) arching the foot. These exercises may be performed isometrically or isotonically.

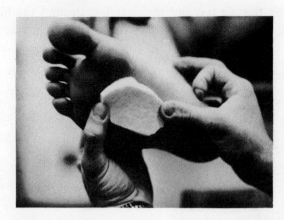

Figure 10-7

Strain

The most common foot strain is of the achilles tendon. There will be pain along the achilles tendon when the toes are brought up toward the leg and sometimes when the toes are pushed away from the leg. There may also be swelling, tenderness, discoloration, and inability to move well.

Strain of the achilles tendon is caused by a strain or blow which causes the tendon to go past its normal range of movement.

Strain of the achilles tendon is best prevented by strengthening the calf muscles and by frequently stretching the back of the leg.

Strain of the achilles tendon is immediately treated by applying cold packs for approximately 30 minutes. Then put a felt pad in the heel area of the athlete's shoe and have him elevate his leg when he gets to his room. Next day apply heat. Tape the achilles tendon to shorten its movement. Figure 10-8 shows how to apply the tape for restricting the achilles tendon range of movement. Have the athlete lie face down on a table. Next place a pillow or pad under the front of his leg so that his toes are pointed away from his leg. With one-and-a-half inch tape, start at the ball of the foot and come up over the heel to the base of the calf muscle. Next start a piece of tape on top of the foot at the ball of the foot, come under the foot, up over the heel, and up the side of the leg to a place even with the first strip of tape. Repeat the procedure on the opposite side of the foot. You should then apply approximately three or four more strips of tape in each of the directions described above.

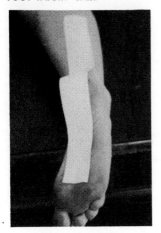
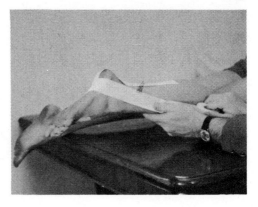

Figure 10-8

Tenosynovitis

Tenosynovitis is an inflammation or irritation of any of the tendons in the foot. There will be pain when the foot moves. You may sometimes be able to feel the roughness of the tendon sheath when the tendon moves.

Tenosynovitis is caused by a blow, bruise, pressure, the athlete's changing sports, or the athlete's not being in shape.

Tenosynovitis is treated and rehabilitated with frequent applications of heat and hot packs. For tenosynovitis of the achilles tendon, immobilize the foot by applying the taping method described in Figure 10-8 on page 203. For tenosynovitis in the foot region, apply tape under the foot with a slight lifting motion and attach it on top of the foot (Figure 10-9).

In all cases of tenosynovitis, place a sponge rubber pad in the athlete's shoe. At all times keep the foot snugly bandaged with a wrap over the tape. The physician may sometimes apply a splint to limit foot movement. He will also attach the splint so that it can be removed for heat treatments for the foot.

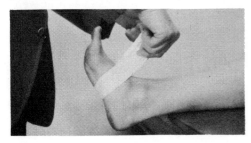

Figure 10-9

11

Arm Injury Care

The arm is divided into the upper arm containing the humerus and the lower arm containing the radius and ulna.

EXAMINATION

When the athlete experiences arm problems, you should (a) make a visual inspection of the upper and lower arm to detect any bleeding, discoloration, obvious deformity, or swelling; (b) feel the arm to learn if there are any unusual protrusions or indentations; and (c) use the following manual tests to determine point of injury when there is no obvious deformity or fracture.

1. Have the athlete bring his lower arm palm up so that it forms a right angle with his upper arm. Next place your hand on his palm and exert downward pressure as he tries to bring his lower arm to his body. This movement will detect damage to the biceps muscle.
2. Have the athlete bring his arm down to the same position described above. Place your hand under his hand and exert upward pressure as he tries to straighten his arm. This movement will detect damage to the triceps muscle.
3. Have the athlete use the same starting position described above. Next have him turn his thumb up and grasp your hand as if he were shaking it. Then have him turn his thumb first inward and then outward. This movement will detect damage to the forearm muscles.

TREATMENT

The above examination procedure will usually identify one or more of the following arm problems: contusion, cut, fracture, or strain.

Contusion

Contusion of the arm is a frequent occurrence in athletics because of the exposed nature of the upper and lower arm. Contusion of the upper arm most frequently occurs on the outer surface midway between the shoulder and elbow joints. Contusion of the lower arm most frequently occurs on the little finger side. There will be localized soreness, swelling, pain on movement, and sometimes loss of movement.

Contusion of the upper and lower arm is caused by blows on the area when the athlete is hit or hits someone or something.

Contusion of the upper and lower arm may be prevented by application of pads.

Contusion of the upper and lower arm is immediately treated with cold and compression. If there is immediate swelling, you should have the athlete's arm X-rayed to check for a fracture. When no fracture is present, next day apply heat, massage, and hot packs.

Contusion of the upper and lower arm is rehabilitated by frequent applications of heat, massage, and the exercises described later.

Cuts

Cuts on the upper or lower arm may occur at anytime. Fortunately, most of the cuts are minor but must be immediately treated to prevent infection. Usually, there will be torn skin and surrounding tissue as well as bleeding. Often there will be pain.

Cuts are caused when the athlete's arm hits a sharp object.

Cuts may be prevented by clearing the playing area of all extraneous objects. The athlete may also prevent his arm from being cut by wearing long sleeved jerseys and protective padding when there is a possibility he may be falling on sharp objects.

Cuts on the arm are immediately treated by lengthwise washing of the wound to remove all foreign matter. After you have thoroughly cleaned the cut, apply ice along with compression to stop the bleeding. Be certain that the bleeding is not from an artery indicated by spurting blood flow. Should the artery be severed, apply direct pressure, elevate the arm, and immediately transport the athlete to a hospital.

Cuts of the arm are rehabilitated by strict adherence to cleanliness. When the athlete participates, the cut area must be protected with a pad.

Fracture

Fracture of the upper or lower arm bones will usually result in localized tenderness, pain, swelling, limitation of movement and deformity. In extreme cases, there may be bleeding, broken skin, and bone fragments through the skin.

Fracture of the arm is caused by blows to the arm or falls. Sometimes a severe sprain or strain will result in a fracture.

Fracture may be prevented by strengthening the arm muscles with the exercises described later. Teaching of proper falling, blocking, and tackling techniques will also help. Oftentimes, protective pads will absorb enough of the shock to prevent a fracture.

Fracture of the arm is treated by immobilizing the upper or lower arm with splints and transportation to a physician.

The upper arm fracture is splinted as follows: Place the athlete's upper arm against his chest so that his forearm is diagonally across his chest with his fingers touching his shoulder. Have someone hold his forearm in this position. Next apply two short splints (rolled up newspaper or magazines will suffice) on the inside and outside of the arm so that they extend slightly below the elbow. Then place a sling on the forearm and support it around the neck. Secure the upper arm against the athlete's side toward the chest with bandages. Figure 11-1 illustrates the upper arm splint.

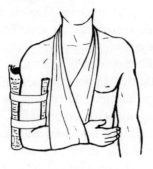

Figure 11-1

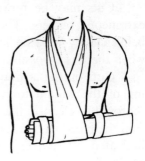

Figure 11-2

The lower arm fracture is splinted as follows: Place the athlete's arm in a palms downward position (normal position). Next apply and secure splints on the top and bottom surface of the arm so that the splints extend past the fingers and the elbow joint. Then place the athlete's arm in a sling. Figure 11-2 shows how to splint the lower arm.

Strain

Strain of the arm affects any of the muscles of the upper or lower arm. There will be severe pain, sometimes discoloration, swelling, localized tenderness, and limitation of movement.

Strain of the upper or lower arm is caused when the muscles are forced or stretched beyond their normal range of motion. Inadequate warmup may also contribute to strain.

Strain of the upper or lower arm may be prevented by strengthening and stretching exercises and by properly warming up the arm muscles.

Strain of the upper or lower arm is immediately treated with cold packs. It is good to place the arm in a sling overnight to assure rest. Next day apply heat, massage, and the exercises described below.

Strain of the arm is rehabilitated by adherence to the treatment procedures outlined above.

EXERCISES

Isometric Exercises

The following isometric exercises are performed twice daily for eight seconds.

The exercise for the biceps muscle is administered as follows: Have the athlete bend his elbow so that his lower arm palm up forms a right angle with his upper arm. Place one hand in his palm and with your other hand stabilize his elbow. Then apply downward pressure as he tries to bend his elbow (Figure 5-18).

The exercise for the triceps muscle is administered as follows: Have the athlete bend his elbow so that his lower arm palm up forms a right angle with his upper arm. Place one hand under the back of his hand and with your other hand stabilize his elbow. Then apply upward pressure as he tries to straighten his elbow (Figure 5-19).

The exercise for the forearm muscle is administered as follows: Have the athlete bend his elbow so that his lower arm thumb up forms a right angle with his upper arm. Then grasp his hand as if you were shaking it and apply resistive pressure as he tries to turn his palm in and as he tries to turn his palm out (Figure 5-20).

Isotonic Exercises

Each of the following isotonic exercises is performed according to the directions described on page 65.

The exercise for the biceps muscle is administered as follows: Have the athlete sit on a table and grasp a weight so his palm is up. Then have him bend and straighten his arm without changing the position of his palm.

The exercise for the triceps muscle is administered as follows: Have the athlete lie face down on a table so that his elbow is at the edge of the table. He then grasps a weight so that his palm is toward his feet and straightens his elbow to full extension and returns the weight to its original starting position.

The exercise for the forearm muscles is administered as follows: Have the athlete sit at a table so that his lower arm forms a right angle with his upper arm and is supported by the table. His wrist should extend approximately 12 inches over the edge. Then with his palm up have him grasp a weight and first turn his palm down and then up.

12

Hand, Finger, and Thumb Injury Care

HAND INJURIES

The hand is defined as the area between the wrist and knuckles. Injuries which occur to the hand area include abrasion, contusion, cut, fracture, puncture, and ruptured blood vessel.

Abrasion

Hand abrasion is the tearing off of the upper layer or layers of skin resulting in bleeding or lymph drainage. Generally, there will be slight pain and localized soreness.

Hand abrasion is caused when the athlete scrapes his hand against a hard, sharp object.

Hand abrasion may be prevented by having the athlete wear hand pads.

Hand abrasion is treated and rehabilitated according to the procedures outlined in Chapter 3.

Contusion

Hand contusion is common in most contact sports. When hit, the hand will usually swell very quickly, and the athlete will experience pain.

Hand contusion is caused by a direct blow on the hand when the athlete hits someone or something or when another athlete steps on his hand.

Hand contusion may be prevented by having the athlete wear protective hand pads.

Hand contusion is treated with immediate application of ice and a compression bandage to reduce swelling. Next day apply heat and a hot pack. Be sure you provide protection for the injured hand (Figure 12-1) when the athlete participates. Do not allow the athlete to participate until he has regained full range of motion in his hand.

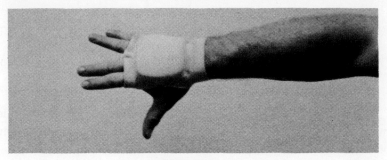

Figure 12-1

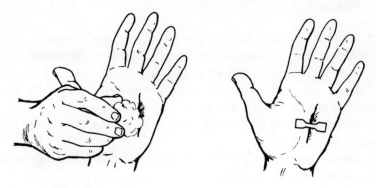

Figure 12-2　　　　　　　　　　　Figure 12-3

Cut

Hand cut involves a wound to the back or palm of the hand. There will be profuse bleeding, localized pain and tenderness, and sometimes loss of function.

Hand cut is caused when the athlete strikes his hand against a sharp object or when he is stepped on by an athlete who has a defective cleat. In baseball, a baserunner can slide into the athlete's hand and cause a severe cut.

Hand cut is rather hard to prevent. However, it can be reduced by keeping sharp objects off of or away from the playing area.

Hand cuts are treated by immediately stopping the blood flow with direct pressure on the cut or an ice application. As soon as the blood flow is stopped, clean the wound by washing it with soap and water in a lengthwise manner (Figure 12-2). If the cut is very deep, apply a butterfly bandage (Figure 12-3) and take the athlete to a physician for sutures.

Hand cuts are rehabilitated by adhering to cleanliness procedures and by protecting the hand during competition.

Fracture

Hand fracture is a break of one or more of the five bones which make up the hand. There will be deformity, swelling, and loss of function. Generally, one of the knuckles will be shorter than the others. There will also be a definite grating (rubbing together) of the bones when you feel the hand area.

Hand fracture is caused by a direct blow to the hand when the athlete strikes an object or when his hand is stepped on by another athlete.

Hand fracture is somewhat difficult to prevent. It is best to provide protective hand guards for contact sports.

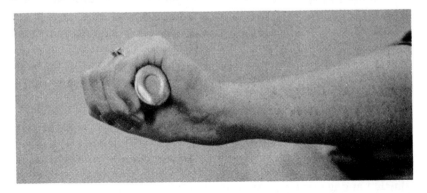

Figure 12-4

Hand fracture is treated by splinting the hand. Figure 12-4 illustrates a method for splinting a hand fracture. Place a gauze roll or elastic bandage in the athlete's palm and have him hold it in place with his fingers. Then starting at his wrist, wrap the entire hand with an elastic wrap. As you apply the wrap, apply firm even pressure. Next place the athlete's arm in a sling, provide ice packs on the hand, and transport the athlete to a physician. When in doubt always have the hand X-rayed before you decide the hand is not fractured. All other treatment is done by the physician.

Puncture

Hand puncture involves a small hole in the hand. There will usually be pain, some swelling, little bleeding, and sometimes discoloration.

Hand punctures are caused when the athlete strikes his hand against a round, sharp object or when he is stepped on by another athlete's cleats.

Hand puncture may be prevented by the athlete's wearing protective hand pads.

Hand puncture is treated by thoroughly cleaning the wound with soap and water. Next apply an antiseptic to the wound. Then have the physician examine the wound to make sure it is clean. It is imperative that you make sure the athlete has had tetanus shots.

Ruptured Blood Vessel

Hand contusion often is accompanied by a ruptured blood vessel. There will be a protruding knot on the contused area, and it will feel spongy. Generally, there will be some pain and sometimes there may be loss of function.

Ruptured blood vessel is caused by a direct blow on the hand when the athlete hits an object or when his hand is stepped on.

Ruptured blood vessel may be prevented by having the athlete wear hand pads.

Ruptured blood vessel is treated by placing a sponge rubber or felt pad over the protrusion. For best results make the pad slightly larger than the protrused area. Then strap the pad in place with an elastic bandage or tape. As soon as you have secured the pad, apply ice packs and transport the athlete to a physician.

FINGER AND THUMB INJURIES

The fingers include the 12 bones and the thumb two bones which articulate with the hand bone. Finger and thumb injuries with which you should be familiar include blood under nail, contusion, dislocation, fracture, laceration, mallet finger (baseball finger), and sprain.

Blood Under Nail

Blood under the nail is an accumulation of blood which becomes trapped under the nail. There will be bleeding, swelling, pain, and tenderness.

Blood under the nail is caused when the athlete's finger is stepped on or when his finger or thumb is hit or he hits his finger or thumb against a hard object.

Blood under the nail is rather difficult to prevent.

Blood under the nail is treated by having the athlete place his injured finger or thumb in a container of ice water for approximately 30 to 45 minutes to stop bleeding. You then relieve the pressure on the nail by releasing the trapped blood. There are essentially two ways of releasing blood from under the nail.

1. Apply an antiseptic to the nail and its surrounding area. Next take a sharp scalpel or some other very sharp instrument and drill a hole in the nail. You obtain much better results when you heat the point of the sharp instrument. If you have no scalpel or other sharp instrument, you can obtain good results by straightening a paper clip and heating it until it is red-hot. Then with gentle pressure slowly push the paper clip through the nail. Do not worry about burning the underlying finger tissue for the blood will cool the paper clip when it comes in contact with it.

2. Blood under the nail which is located near the end of the fingernail may be released by slipping a sharp, flat instrument under the end of the nail and gently lifting the end of the nail.

Contusion

Contusion of the fingers or thumb is a bruise which often

affects the bone covering. There will be immediate, sharp pain, tenderness, swelling, some loss of function, and discoloration.

Contusion of the fingers or thumb is caused by a direct blow to the fingers or thumb when the athlete hits a hard object, is stepped on, or when a hard object hits his fingers or thumb.

Contusion of the fingers or thumb may be prevented by wearing protective finger guards or gloves when the athlete participates in a sport conducive to blows to the finger or thumb area.

Contusion of the finger or thumb is treated by immediately immersing the finger or thumb in an ice filled container for approximately 30 minutes. Next day apply heat to improve circulation. For competition, you should tape the injured finger to an adjoining finger and provide protective equipment.

Contusion of the finger is rehabilitated by close adherence to treatment procedures. You have to be very diligent during the rehabilitative process since there is not an overabundance of blood to the fingers.

Dislocation

Dislocation of the finger or thumb may involve any of the joints within the finger or thumb. There will be immediate loss of function, deformity, swelling, and pain. Generally, the finger is dislocated at the first or second joint in such a way that it resembles a step (Figure 12-5). The thumb most often is dislocated at its jointure with the hand.

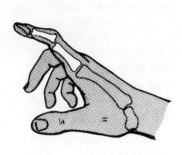

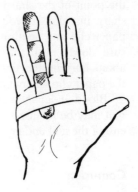

Figure 12-5   Figure 12-6

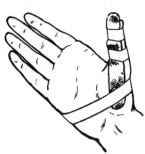

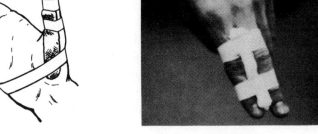

Figure 12-7   Figure 12-8

Dislocation of the finger or thumb is caused when the end of the athlete's finger or thumb is hit or when the athlete jams his finger or thumb against an immoveable object.

Dislocation of the finger or thumb may be prevented by teaching the athlete to keep his fingers and thumb together as much as possible. When the athlete is catching a baseball he should always have his bare hand closed until the ball is in the glove.

Dislocation of the finger or thumb is treated by the physician. You should never attempt to reduce the dislocation since there is always the possibility of a fracture being present. After the physician reduces the dislocation, the athlete's finger is then splinted for approximately ten days or until the physician tells you to remove the splint. During this ten day period, the athlete should keep his hand elevated as much as possible. The finger splint (Figure 12-6) and the thumb splint (Figure 12-7) can be made from a tongue depressor or any other straight, flat, hard object. It should be padded with gauze and should extend below the base of the finger or thumb and past the end. The splint is held in place with tape or gauze wrap. Remember that the splint's major function is to prevent movement.

Dislocation of the finger or thumb rehabilitation begins when the physician gives permission. During this phase, you apply heat and request the athlete to move the finger or thumb through a full range of motion. When the athlete participates, the dislocated finger should be taped to its adjoining finger so that the uninjured finger acts as a splint. If you do not want the finger to move, you should completely cover the two fingers with tape. For some movement in the finger, you apply strips of one-inch tape between knuckles and the first joint and between the first and second joints (Figure 12-8).

The thumb may be taped at least two ways depending on the severity of the injury. Figure 12-9 shows how to tape the thumb for restriction of its movement in all directions. Prepare the area to be taped by spraying with skin toughener. Next apply one-inch tape around the wrist, under the thumb, and back over the wrist. Continue this procedure until you have immobilized the thumb. Figure 12-10 shows how to tape the thumb to keep it from being hyperextended. Take one-inch tape and form a closed loop. Next place the loop so that it rests on the first joint of the thumb and the base of the forefinger. Then tape the loop in its center so that it will fit snugly against the forefinger and thumb. An alternate way of strapping the thumb for prevention of hyperextension consists of taking a piece of one-inch tape and wrapping it around the palm and back of the hand just below the jointure of the fingers with the hand and around the thumb. Next tape the loop together between the fingers and thumb so that the tape will fit snugly against the hand and finger.

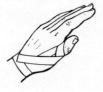

Figure 12-9

Figure 12-10

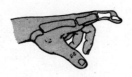

Figure 12-11

Fracture

Fracture of the finger or thumb may occur on any of its parts. The fracture may vary from a hairline crack to a compound fracture. There will be tenderness over the fracture site, possible deformity, swelling, pain, and in cases of compound fracture possible bleeding from broken tissue.

Fracture of the finger or thumb is caused by a direct blow on the finger or thumb. A severe sprain of the finger or thumb may also result in a chip fracture.

Fracture of the finger or thumb is rather hard to prevent. Make sure the athlete knows that he should keep his bare fingers and thumb closed whenever he catches an object in a glove.

Fracture of the finger or thumb is treated by making a correct evaluation of the injury. The best method is to gently pull the finger or thumb and then move it from side to side as you feel for bone movement, tap with your finger over the tender area on the athlete's finger or thumb, and tap on the end of the athlete's finger or thumb. Next you should splint the finger or thumb as illustrated in Figures 12-6 and 12-7. All other treatment is under the physician's supervision.

Fracture of the finger or thumb rehabilitation begins when the athlete is released by the physician. You then follow the same procedures outlined earlier for finger or thumb dislocation.

Laceration

Laceration of the finger or thumb is a jagged tear of the skin and surrounding tissue. There will be bleeding, pain, and sometimes a numbness.

Laceration of the finger or thumb is caused when the athlete strikes his finger or thumb against a sharp object or when the athlete has his finger or thumb stepped on by another athlete.

Laceration of the finger or thumb may be prevented by keeping all extraneous materials off the playing areas and by making sure all the athlete's shoe cleats are in good condition.

Lacerations of the finger or thumb are treated by the physician who will determine whether sutures are needed. The only thing you should do is clean the finger with soap and water and wrap with a non-adhering bandage.

Mallet Finger (Baseball Finger)

Mallet finger is a fracture of the first joint of the finger in which the tendon is pulled away from the bone. The first joint will be in a flexed position (Figure 12-11). There will be pain, swelling, and limitation of movement.

Mallet finger is caused when the athlete's finger is hit on the end by a thrown object or when the athlete hits the end of his finger against something.

Mallet finger may be prevented by teaching the athlete to keep his bare fingers closed until the ball hits the glove.

Mallet finger is treated by the physician.

Sprain

Sprain of the finger or thumb is a result of the finger's being forced beyond its normal range of movement. There will be pain, swelling, discoloration, and some limitation of movement.

Sprain of the finger or thumb is caused when the athlete's finger or thumb is hit on the end and pushed backward past its normal range. The athlete may also twist the finger or thumb at its jointure when he catches his finger or thumb on another athlete's equipment.

Sprain of the finger or thumb is best prevented through the athlete's own efforts.

Sprain of the finger or thumb is treated by immediately immersing the athlete's finger or thumb in a bucket of ice water for 30 to 45 minutes. Next splint the finger or thumb, as illustrated in Figures 12-6 and 12-7 for one or two days. Then start heat treatments by having the athlete soak his hand in hot water baths.

Sprain of the finger or thumb is rehabilitated by following treatment procedures. The objective is to return the finger or thumb as near its normal size as possible. Do not be alarmed, however, if the sprained finger does not return to its normal size. Tape the sprained finger to an uninjured finger when the athlete competes. Tape the sprained thumb as illustrated in Figures 12-8 or 12-9.

13

Heat Related Problems

Excessive environmental heat often results in heat cramps, heat exhaustion, or heat stroke. The most common heat problem found in athletics is heat exhaustion. Heat problems frequently affect the athlete who has been rather physically inactive or who has worked in an air conditioned office during the summer months. An athlete who reports overweight is especially susceptible to heat related problems.

HEAT CRAMPS

Heat cramps are the involuntary contractions of the muscles. Heat cramps usually affect the abdominal and leg muscles. There will be severe muscle spasms, pain, and loss of function in the case of the legs.

Heat cramps are caused by an inadequate salt balance due to profuse sweating in a hot, humid environment.

Heat cramps may be prevented by making sure the athlete includes extra salt in his diet. It is estimated that the average athlete must take in approximately one-half ounce of salt (approximately 3 or 4 level teaspoons) during the day to off-set heat cramps. This needed salt requirement can be adequately met by the athlete's liberally salting his food.

Heat cramps are treated by applying firm pressure to the affected area. In the case of a leg, you just grab the spasm with both hands and squeeze as hard as you can. As soon as you have the spasm stopped, you should then apply warm, wet towels. During the application of the towels, you should also have the athlete drink salt water solution consisting of one-half teaspoon per half-glass of water. A good guide is to make sure the salt can be tasted.

Heat cramps are rehabilitated by adhering to the treatment procedure for approximately 24 hours. You then must maintain a close watch on the athlete to make sure the cramps do not become chronic.

HEAT EXHAUSTION

Heat exhaustion (heat prostration) is an imbalance of salt in the system leading to severe dehydration. There will be extreme fatigue, muscle spasms, nausea, pale, moist skin, abdominal pain, normal pulse, and prostration. The physiological result is that the cardiovascular (heat-lung system) limitations have been exceeded resulting in inadequate circulation.

Heat exhaustion may be prevented by limiting physical exertion when there is a hot, humid day, providing adequate salt in the diet, wearing light, well-ventilated clothing, and acclimating the athletes to the weather conditions before making them perform excessively hard physical work.

Heat exhaustion is immediately treated by placing the athlete in a backlying position in a shaded or cool area. If he is not sick at his stomach, you may give the athlete a cool salt water solution. The important thing for you to do is call a physician and watch the athlete for signs of circulatory failure denoted by pale, cool skin especially in the finger and toe areas. Be sure to keep the athlete quiet during the treatment phase.

HEAT STROKE

Heat stroke is a very high body temperature resulting in unconsciousness, hot, dry, flushed skin, high fever, muscle spasms, dizziness, weakness, convulsions, and rapid pulse. It is essentially a failure of the heat regulating system in the body.

Heat stroke is caused when the athlete does hard physical work during hot weather with a temperature range from 90 to 100 degrees. Generally, the condition occurs when the athlete is exposed over a period of time to the hot rays of the sun. Heat stroke may also occur when there is either high or low humidity.

Heat stroke may be prevented by not making the athletes perform excessive physical exertion during the hot hours of the day. It is especially important for the athletes not to participate in heavy pads or clothing when the temperature is excessively high. You should also be certain the athletes are gradually acclimated to the environment in which they must participate.

Heat stroke is treated by immediate recognition of the injury. You can tell that heat stroke instead of heat exhaustion is present by observing the condition of the athlete's skin. In heat stroke, his skin will always be hot and flushed and his pulse will be fast. Send someone to call the physician. Then start progressively lowering the athlete's temperature by placing the athlete in a cool bath or by applying ice packs or ice spray to his skin. Be certain that you do not bring the temperature down too quickly or the athlete may go into shock and death. This is about all you can do until the physician arrives. He will then take over treatment.

14

The Athlete and Drugs

The knowledge that drug abuse has invaded the athletic sanctuaries presents additional problems for coaches. To meet this problem head-on, you must become familiar with the ways to identify drug abuse and what to do when you suspect abuse. These steps are necessary in order to alleviate a major problem before it causes harm to your program.

WAYS TO IDENTIFY DRUG ABUSERS

There are numerous behavioral clues which will help you identify the athlete who abuses drugs. These include:

1. The athlete's life style undergoing a drastic change, especially when the new life style becomes his pattern of life.
2. The athlete's demonstrating a radical change in his personal appearance. Be aware of whether or not the athlete has just started wearing long sleeved shirts exclusively.
3. The athlete's making a radical change in his mental and physical performance. Be especially alert when the athlete experiences loss of memory, confusion, or incoherence for no apparent reason.
4. The athlete's becoming overly-secretive about himself. You should always become alert when the athlete seems suspicious of your dealings with him regardless of the nature of these activities.

5. The athlete's sudden need for money. He will usually demonstrate this need for money by either stealing or borrowing money or pawnable items from his friends.
6. The athlete's frequent habitation of closets, storage rooms, parked cars (alone), or inaccessible areas.
7. The athlete's association with other persons who are known drug abusers. Special note of this association should be made if the athlete was not formerly friendly with these associates.
8. The athlete's wearing sunglasses at odd times. His primary motive is to protect his eyes from the light and prevent you from noticing the condition of his eyes.
9. The athlete's frequent outbursts of temper for no apparent reason.
10. The athlete's deviating from his normal speech pattern by using slang terms connected with the drug abuser, i.e., cooker, fix, speed, grass, freak, spike, etc.
11. The athlete's experiencing frequent drowsy spells.
12. The athlete's exhibiting undue excitement patterns.
13. The athlete's demonstrating a distasteful attitude toward authority or toward those persons he previously admired.
14. The athlete's having in his possession any form of drug or a spoon with a bent handle or bottle cap, ball of cotton, syringe or eye dropper, or a hypodermic needle.

CLASSIFICATION OF DRUGS

Should you note any or a combination of the above physical or social symptoms of drug abuse, you must then determine what type of drugs the athlete might be using. Basically, drugs are classified as depressants, hallucinogens, stimulants, or vapors.

DEPRESSANTS

Depressants are drugs which sedate the individual by acting on the central nervous system. Medically, they are used to treat anxiety, high blood pressure, and tension. When abused, depressants may cause drowsiness, decrease imagination, judgment, and self-control, cause a loss of a sense of time and space, cause a confused state of mind, cause a feeling of well-being, cause depression, or cause irritability. Common depressants include barbiturates and narcotics.

Barbiturates

Barbiturates are chemical compounds which induce sleep, sedate, or induce a hypnotic state. They are habit forming and when abused will cause the athlete to have any or all of the following symptoms.

1. He may have all the signs of being drunk, except there will be no alcohol odor.
2. He may be relaxed, overly-sociable, and good-humored, but slow to react.
3. He may be sluggish, gloomy, and quarrelsome.
4. He may stagger, be thick-tongued, and be sleepy.
5. He may lapse into a coma which if left untreated will cause death.

Commonly abused barbiturates follow:

1. Amytal is called blues, blue heaven, blue birds, blue devils, or amabarbital solution. Generally, you will be able to identify amytal by its blue color and its capsule form.
2. Luminal is called purple hearts, phenobarbital, or truth serum. It is a phenobarbital capsule which might be yellow, yellow and white, white with purple strip, or light and dark orange, depending on the manufacturers.
3. Nembutal is called yellow jackets, yellows, nimbie, nimby, nemmies, or phenobarbital solution. It is generally in a capsule and yellow in color.
4. Seconal is called reds, red birds, red devils, seggy, seccy, pinks, or secobarbital sodium. It may be red or pink in color and is usually in capsule form.
5. Trinal is called rainbow, double trouble, tooies, or amobarbital plus secobarbital. It is in capsule form and may be either orange, light purple, or blue-black and white.

Narcotics

Narcotics are derived from opium, and their function is to induce sleep or a stupor for the purpose of relieving pain. They are addictive, and when abused will cause the athlete to appear drowsy, to show signs of deep intoxication, and to have constricted pupils of the eye that will not respond to light.

Generally, the athlete who abuses narcotics will no longer be a member of the team, for he will not be able to function in an ordered environment. However, it is imperative for you to notice incidents which will indicate potential narcotic abusers on your team. These clues include:

1. The presence of cough medicine or paregoric bottles in the dressing room area or in wastebaskets around the dressing room or playing area.
2. The presence of cough medicine or paregoric on the athlete's breath.
3. The traces of white powder around the athlete's nostrils.
4. The athlete's nostrils being constantly red and inflamed.
5. The presence of needle marks on the inner surface of the athlete's arm at the elbow.
6. The presence of narcotic equipment such as a blackened spoon with a bent handle, a bottle cap, small ball of cotton, syringe or eye-dropper, and a hypodermic needle. Usually this equipment will be on the athlete or else hidden in a private place which is easily accessible to the athlete.

Commonly abused narcotics are:

1. Codeine is called schoolboy and is primarily used to ease pain and to alleviate coughing. It is taken orally and if abused will cause drowsiness and addiction. It is widely used in cough medicines. In its natural state, codeine is an odorless white crystal or crystalline powder which is dispensed either in tablet form or in a liquid solution.
2. Heroin is called "H," horse, scat, junk, hard stuff, Harry, joy, scag, or powder. It is produced from morphine and in its natural state is a grayish-brown color; however, you will most often see it when it has been diluted for sale, at which time it is either white or off-white. Heroin is either sniffed or injected, but for best results, it must be injected. Therefore, you should note any needle marks or scar tissue on the body of the athlete. You might also be cognizant of burns about the nose or mouth area, and be especially alert if you have an athlete who has frequently inflamed nostrils.
3. Meperidine, a synthetic morphine-like drug, is often referred to as demorol. Its purpose is to relieve pain, and it is ingested orally or by injection. The athlete, when he abuses this drug, will become

excited, tremor, and sometimes convulse. It is obtained in tablet, capsule, or liquid form.

4. Morphine is a derivative of opium with a primary purpose of relieving pain. It will cause drowsiness, stupor, and pupils of the eye will not react to light. It may be taken orally or by injection. It is most commonly found in liquid form.

HALLUCINOGENS

Hallucinogens are drugs often called psychedelics, which produce sensations of a distortion of time, space, sound, and color by affecting the central nervous system. An athlete under the influence of a hallucinogen will exhibit one or more of the following symptoms:

1. He will sit or lie in a dream-like or trance-like state.
2. He may become fearful or experience a degree of tremor, causing him to try an escape from the crowd.
3. He may experience a drastic change in his mood or personality.
4. He may experience a sensation of being outside his body.

Hallucinogens may be in tablet, capsule or leaf form, but they are most commonly found in a liquid form. Because of the liquid base, hallucinogens are sometimes accidentally ingested. Therefore, you should be aware of what company your athletes keep. At any time the athlete acts unusual, have him examined by a physician.

Commonly abused hallucinogens include:

1. LSD is derived from ergot, which is found on wheat, rye, or other grasses as well as the morning glory. LSD is ingested orally and may be found in capsule, tablet, or liquid form. LSD users will react differently to the drug, and the user will usually know that his reactions are drug induced.
2. Marijuana is referred to as pot, weed, hemp, grass, hash, rope, kif, or stuff. It is usually smoked and is distinguishable by its rope-burning-like smell. The drug, when lightly used, is hard to detect, but as the athlete smokes, he will become animated and then gradually become sleepy. At all stages, he will have dilated pupils of the eye. Marijuana is typically smoked in a group situation, and the cigarette can be identified as a double thickness of brownish or off-white paper. The cigarette is smaller than a regular cigarette,

with the ends being twisted. Additionally, the marijuana cigarette sometimes contains seeds and stems and is somewhat greener than regular tobacco. Usually, the marijuana user will have an odor of burnt rope on his clothes and breath.

3. STP is referred to as dom, serenity, tranquility, or peace. Chemically, STP is related to mescaline and amphetamine. An athlete under the influence of STP will possibly experience nausea, sweating, tremors, blurred vision, multiple images, visual and auditory hallucinations, vibration of objects, enhancement of detail, and distortions of time. STP can be obtained in tablet or capsule form.

STIMULANTS

Stimulants act on the central nervous system to produce excitation, alertness, and wakefulness. Medically, it is used to treat mild depressive states, overweight, and narcolepsy (excessive desire to sleep). Stimulants are obtainable in capsule, tablet, or liquid form. General signs of stimulant abuse are excessive activity, irritability, and nervousness. Additionally, the athlete may have dilated pupils of the eye, which do not react to light.

Commonly abused stimulants include the amphetamine family. Amphetamine abuse causes the athlete to show one or more of the following symptoms:

1. He may have dry mucous membranes of the mouth and nose with resulting bad breath.
2. He may lick his lips because of the drying effect of the amphetamine.
3. He may frequently and vigorously rub his nose.
4. He may talk incessantly about any subject.
5. He may go long periods of time without sleep or food and brag about it.
6. He may have dilated eye pupils which will not react to light.
7. He may hallucinate.
8. He may be restless.
9. He may have tremors.

Commonly used amphetamines follow:

1. Benzedrine may be called bennie, benzies, peaches, roses,

hearts, cartwheels, or amphetamine sulphate. It is obtainable in capsule or pill form. Primarily, it is used to prevent sleep. It is ingested orally or by an injection.

2. Dexedrine may be called hearts, organes, dexies, footballs, or dextroamphetamine sulphate. It is used to suppress appetite and to prevent sleep and fatigue. It may be ingested orally or by injection.

3. Methedrine may be called crystal, meth, speed, hydrochloride, businessman's trip, syndrox, desoxyn, or bombites. It is used to prevent sleep, fatigue, and to suppress appetite. It may be ingested orally or by injection.

VAPORS

Vapor abuse is the deliberate inhalation of a solvent, most often glue, for the express purpose of getting high. When the athlete inhales vapors, he will exhibit the following:

1. He may retain an odor of the inhaled substance on his breath or clothing.
2. He may have inflamed membranes in the mouth and nose, as well as excessive nasal secretions.
3. He may have red, watery eyes.
4. He may appear intoxicated.
5. He may lack muscular control.
6. He may complain of double vision, ringing ears, vivid dreams, and hallucinations.
7. He may appear to be in a drowsy or stupor state.
8. He may be unconscious, especially when he uses an excessive amount.
9. He may have in his possession or in or near his locker, plastic or paper bags and rags or handkerchiefs containing dried plastic cement or other substance of a vapor nature.

Common vapors which are abused include glue, ether, chloroform, gasoline, lighter fluid, refrigerants, carbon tetrochloride, paint thinner, shellac, and kerosene.

WAYS TO PREVENT DRUG ABUSE

There are a number of ways you might be able to prevent drug abuse among your athletes. First, you should present the facts, as they are known, concerning drug abuse. You should at all costs avoid "preaching" to your athletes. Factual drug information is best provided by the local narcotics bureau of the police department.

Second, you should have an established policy (preferably written) concerning drug problems on the team. The primary parts of this policy should include procedures for handling suspected drug abusers and procedures for emergency handling of drug cases.

Third, you must always be aware of the amount and type of medication prescribed for your athletes. Additionally, be certain the person who is handling your drugs is a reliable individual. You might also check, when you see an athlete with pills or other medications, for a prescription.

Fourth, you should carefully screen individuals who are constantly around the dressing room or playing area. Be alert when their actions seem unusual.

Fifth, you should have meetings, when it appears necessary, with law enforcement personnel to assure yourself that your athletes have not been seen with known drug abusers or engaged in illicit drug activity.

WHAT TO DO WHEN DRUGS ARE ABUSED

The way you handle problems of suspected drug abuse will vary; however, there are a few guide lines you might find helpful.

1. You must be certain that a drug abuse problem actually exists.
2. You must accept a responsible role in helping counsel with the athlete, parents, educators, and law enforcement personnel. Your actions here can make or break the athlete. Your primary concern must be with the effect drugs have on your team and on the involved athlete. You must never ignore a drug abuse problem, for it will only worsen.
3. You must immediately seek the advice of a physician when the athlete begins to behave in an unusual manner. In this way, you assess the true reason for the athlete's behavior. Moreover, by seeking medical advice and care, you can alleviate the problem before it runs amuck.
4. You must make every effort at your disposal to find the source of drug traffic on your campus or in your town. This course of

action will help to prevent the spread of drug abuse among your athletes.

5. You should establish a good working relationship with law enforcement officials. Seek their advice, be candid about your problems, but be careful in revealing confidential information.

6. You must try to understand and try to help the athlete who has succumbed to the drug habit. If he is one of the lesser stars, you should be unusually considerate. In doing so, you will enhance rapport with your athletes, and thus make it easier for you to recognize problems when they are just beginning.

Appendix

ATHLETIC MEDICAL HISTORY*

Name _____ Age _____

Home Address _____

Parents' Name _____

Telephone Number _____ Religious Preference _____

Family History

	Age	State of Health, If Living	Cause of Death	Age at Death
Father	_____	_____	_____	_____
Mother	_____	_____	_____	_____
Brothers	_____	_____	_____	_____
Sisters	_____	_____	_____	_____
Wife	_____	_____	_____	_____

Who in your family has had: Goiter _____ Diabetes _____

Cancer _____ Tuberculosis _____ Allergies or

Asthma _____ Heart disease at an early age _____

High Blood Pressure _____ Gout _____

Strokes _____ Mental Disorder _____ Convulsions

or Epilepsy _____ Migraine Headaches _____

Personal Habits

Average number of hours sleep _____ Do you frequently

miss breakfast? _____ Eat or drink between meals or at

bedtime? _____ Eat sweets? _____ Drink alcoholic

beverages? _____ How much? _____ Eat too rapidly

or too much _____ Do you regularly or frequently smoke?

_____ Cigarettes _____ Cigars _____

_____

* Used by permission of the University of Florida Division of Intercollegiate
Athletics.

Pipe _____ How many per day? _____ For how
long (years)? _____ Do you exercise regularly? _____
Hobbies _____

Personal Health History

Please check the correct answer following each question:

I. Head Injury

    A. Have you ever been unconscious? Yes _____ No _____

    B. Did this occur while participating in football? Yes _____
       No _____

    C. How long were you unconscious?

                       less than 5 minutes _____
                       less than 15 minutes _____
                       over 15 minutes _____

    D. Were you seen by a physician? Yes _____ No _____

    E. Were you admitted to a hospital or infirmary? Yes _____
       No _____

    F. Were Xrays made? Yes _____ No _____

    G. How long after being unconscious before you were allowed to
       participate in football again?

                       less than 2 days _____
                       less than 1 week _____
                       over 1 week _____

    H. Have you ever had a skull fracture? Yes _____ No _____

    I. Have you ever had amnesia (loss of memory) following a head
       injury? Yes _____ No _____

    J. Have you ever had a convulsion? Yes _____ No _____

    K. Do you have frequent headaches? Yes _____ No _____

    L. Have you ever had blurred or double vision? Yes _____

II. Eyes

    A. Do you have absence of one eye? Yes _____ No _____

B. Do you have diminished or abnormal vision? Yes _____
   No _____

C. Do you normally wear glasses? Yes _____ No _____

D. Do you wear contact lenses? Yes _____ No _____

III. Ears

A. Do you have any defect of hearing? Yes _____ No _____

IV. Nose

A. Do you have frequent nose bleed? Yes _____ No _____

B. Have you ever broken your nose? Yes _____ No _____

C. If broken, did you have surgery? Yes _____ No _____

V. Dental

A. Do you have any false teeth or plates? Yes _____ No _____

B. Have you fractured a tooth playing football? Yes _____
   No _____

C. Have you had a tooth knocked-out playing football?
   Yes _____ No _____

D. Have you had more than one tooth knocked-out?
   Yes _____ No _____

E. Did you miss any practice because of the injury? Yes _____
   No _____

F. Do you wear a tooth or mouth protector when playing football?
   Yes _____ No _____

G. Do you think tooth protectors should be required in college as
   they are in high school? Yes _____ No _____

VI. Neck

A. Have you ever sustained a neck injury while playing football?
   Yes _____ No _____

B. Did you have numbness, burning or sharp pain in your arms
   and hands? Yes _____ No _____

C. Did you see a physician? Yes _____ No _____

D. Were Xrays made? Yes _____ No _____

E. Were you in a hospital or Infirmary?   Yes _____ No _____

F. How long did you miss practice following injury?

less than 2 days _____

less than 1 week _____

more than 1 week _____

G. Have you ever worn a "horse collar" because of a neck injury?
Yes _____ No _____

H. If answer to (G) was yes, did the collar reduce the incidence
of neck injury?   Yes _____ No _____

I. Have you been taught to "spear" with your head when you
tackle and block?   Yes _____ No _____

VII. Musculoskeletal

A. Dislocations

1. Have you ever dislocated a joint?   Yes _____ No _____
2. If answer to #1 is yes, please check involved area or areas:
Shoulder _____   Ankle _____
Knee-cap (patella) _____   Finger _____
Knee _____   A-C Sep _____
3. If answer to #1 was yes, has the dislocation occurred more
than once?   Yes _____ No _____
4. Did you see a physician with initial dislocation?
Yes _____ No _____
5. Were Xrays made?   Yes _____ No _____
6. Was the involved area immobilized?   Yes _____
No _____
7. Did you have surgery?   Yes _____ No _____
8. Were you given specific exercises following the injury or
surgery?   Yes _____ No _____

B. Spine

1. Have you ever injured your back?   Yes _____ No _____
2. Have you injured your back more than once?   Yes _____
No _____
3. When did you first have back trouble?

before high school _____

during high school _____

during college _____

4. Did you see a physician?   Yes _____ No _____

5. Were Xrays made?   Yes _____ No _____
6. How long did you miss practice?

less than 2 days _____
less than 1 week _____
more than 1 week _____

7. Were you ever told that you have a spinal defect that has been present since birth?   Yes _____ No _____
8. Were you instructed in special exercises for your back? Yes _____ No _____

C. *Knee*

1. Have you ever had a significant knee injury? Yes _____ No _____
2. When did you first injure your knee?

before high school _____
during high school _____
during college _____

3. Did you see a physician?   Yes _____ No _____
4. Did you have Xrays?   Yes _____ No _____
5. Did you have surgery?   Yes _____ No _____
6. Were you given specific knee exercises following surgery or injury?   Yes _____ No _____
7. How long did you miss practice?

less than 2 days _____
less than 1 week _____
more than 1 week _____

8. Have you had significant injuries to both knees? Yes _____ No _____
9. Have you had surgery on both knees?   Yes _____ No _____
10. Have you had surgery on either knee more than once? Yes _____ No _____
11. If you had a knee injury in college, did this represent a re-injury from high school?   Yes _____ No _____
12. If you had a knee injury in high school, do you think the injury was properly treated?   Yes _____ No _____
13. (a) Does your knee swell?   Yes _____ No _____
    (b) lock?   Yes _____ No _____
    (c) giveaway?   Yes _____ No _____
    (d) feel unstable?   Yes _____ No _____
    (e) hurt following activity?   Yes _____ No _____

D. *Fractures*

1. Have you ever had a broken bone?   Yes _____ No _____

2. If #1 was yes, check involved area
   - (a) Nose _____
   - (b) Face _____
   - (c) Neck _____
   - (d) Back _____
   - (e) Arm _____
   - (f) Forearm _____
   - (g) Ribs _____
   - (h) Hand _____
   - (i) Pelvis _____
   - (j) Thigh _____
   - (k) Leg _____
   - (l) Foot _____
   - (m) Skull _____
   - (n) Clavicle _____

3. If #1 was yes, was the fracture a result of football participation? Yes _____ No _____

4. If yes, was your athletic performance altered following injury? Yes _____ No _____

5. Do you have any residual defect as a result of the fracture? Yes _____ No _____

E. *Myositis Ossificans Traumatica*

1. Have you ever had calcium to form in your thigh or arm following a bad bruise? Yes _____ No _____

2. How much time did you miss from practice?
   - less than 2 days _____
   - less than 1 week _____
   - more than 1 week _____

3. Was the calcium surgically removed? Yes _____ No _____

4. Do you still have trouble as the result of this injury? Yes _____ No _____

F. *Muscle Strain*

1. Have you ever had a bad "Muscle pull" or strain? Yes _____ No _____

2. How much time did you miss from practice?
   - less than 2 days _____
   - less than 1 week _____
   - more than 1 week _____

3. Did the injury recur? Yes _____ No _____

4. More than once? Yes _____ No _____

5. Did the muscle pull occur initially
   - before high school _____
   - during high school _____
   - during college _____

G. *Ankle Sprain*

1. Have you ever sprained your ankle?
   Yes _____ No _____

2. If yes, when did you first sprain your ankle?

before high school _____
during high school _____
during college _____

3. When first sprained was your
ankle taped: Yes _____ No _____
wrapped: Yes _____ No _____
4. Did you see a physician?   Yes _____ No _____
5. Was an Xray made?   Yes _____ No _____
6. Did you have surgery?   Yes _____ No _____
7. Did you have any immobi-
lization?   Yes _____ No _____
8. Have you had recurrent sprains
of the ankle?   Yes _____ No _____
9. Have both ankles been
sprained?   Yes _____ No _____
10. At present do you always tape
or wrap your ankles?   Yes _____ No _____

VIII. Have you ever had or do you have . . .

A. Cardiac

1. High blood pressure   Yes _____ No _____
2. Rheumatic heart disease   Yes _____ No _____
3. Any heart disease since birth
(congenital)   Yes _____ No _____
4. Abnormal heart rate   Yes _____ No _____
5. Palpitation   Yes _____ No _____
6. Heart Murmur   Yes _____ No _____

B. Genitourinary

1. Absence of one kidney   Yes _____ No _____
2. Frequent urinary infection Yes _____ No _____
3. Kidney stone   Yes _____ No _____
4. Blood in urine   Yes _____ No _____

C. Gastrointestinal

1. Frequent diarrhea   Yes _____ No _____
2. Frequent constipation   Yes _____ No _____
3. Peptic ulcer   Yes _____ No _____
4. Pregame stress (nausea,
vomiting, etc.)   Yes _____ No _____
5. Liver infection (hepatitis) Yes _____ No _____
6. Jaundice   Yes _____ No _____

7. Enlarged Spleen   Yes _____ No _____
8. Ruptured Spleen   Yes _____ No _____
9. Hernia   Yes _____ No _____

D. *Skin*

1. Frequent boils   Yes _____ No _____
2. Severe acne   Yes _____ No _____
3. Athlete's foot   Yes _____ No _____
4. "jock itch"   Yes _____ No _____

E. *Miscellaneous Diseases*

1. Diabetes   Yes _____ No _____
2. Polio   Yes _____ No _____
3. Tuberculosis   Yes _____ No _____
4. Asthma   Yes _____ No _____
5. Infectious mononucleosis   Yes _____ No _____
6. Epilepsy   Yes _____ No _____
7. Food allergy   Yes _____ No _____
8. Drug allergy   Yes _____ No _____
9. Pollen allergy   Yes _____ No _____
10. Abnormal bruising   Yes _____ No _____
11. Abnormal bleeding tendency   Yes _____ No _____

F. *Surgery*

1. Appendectomy   Yes _____ No _____
2. Tonsillectomy   Yes _____ No _____
3. Hernia repair   Yes _____ No _____
4. Other surgery   Yes _____ No _____

G. *Heat Disorder*

1. Have you ever had trouble with dehydration (excess loss of salt and water)?   Yes _____ No _____
2. Have you ever had heat stroke?   Yes _____ No _____
3. If answer to #2 is yes, were you hospitalized?   Yes _____ No _____
4. How long did you miss practice?   less than 2 days _____
                                   less than 1 week _____
                                   more than 1 week _____

H. *Immunizations*

1. Have you been immunized against tetanus?   Yes _____ No _____

2. Have you been immunized
against flu?   Yes _____ No _____
3. Have you been immunized
against polio?   Yes _____ No _____

IX. Drug, Food Supplements and Miscellaneous Agents

	Never	Rarely	Occ.	Freq.
A. *Vitamin*				
B. *Wheat germ*				
C. *Bone meal*				
D. *Stimulants* (benzadrine, amphetamine)				
E. *Cigarette*				
F. *Sleeping pills*				
G. *Alcoholic beverages*				
H. *Anabolic agents* (growth stimulators)				

X. Training and conditioning

Check appropriate space which most closely resembles your own training and conditioning program.

A. *Length of training*
1. Some form of training year around   Yes _____ No _____
2. Training 9 months per year   Yes _____ No _____
3. Training 6 months per year   Yes _____ No _____
4. Training 4 months per year   Yes _____ No _____

B. *Training items*
1. Weight lifting   Yes _____ No _____
2. Isometrics   Yes _____ No _____
3. Flexibility exercises   Yes _____ No _____
4. Specific exercises for shoulders   Yes _____ No _____
5. Specific exercises for knees   Yes _____ No _____
6. Specific exercises for back   Yes _____ No _____
7. Reaction training   Yes _____ No _____
8. Endurance training   Yes _____ No _____

XI. *Value of sports*

1. Do you feel that your participation in football has strengthened your character and in other ways made you a better person?

    Yes _____ No _____

2. Would you like your son to play football?

    Yes _____ No _____

---

* Used by permission of the University of Florida Division of Intercollegiate Athletics.

NAME _____ / _____
Born _____ / _____
Soc. Sec. #
Home Address:
Home Telephone:

UNIVERSITY OF FLORIDA
Athletic Physical Examination Form*

Doctors: Mark "negatives" c̄ "o". Mark "defects" c̄ "x" and describe (where necessary use "Remarks" section). Where applicable mark the abnormality 1°, 2°, 3°.

School Year	Fall	Fall	Fall	Fall	Fall
1. Wt. / Ht.	/	/	/	/	/
2. Urine - Glucose					
Alb. / S.G. / Micro.					
3. Blood hgb / WBC / hct					
4. Blood Pressure sys. / dia.	sys. / dia.	sys. / dia.	sys. / dia.	sys. / dia.	sys. / dia.
5. Heart Pulse					
Rhythm					
6. Lungs Ausc. Percuss.					
X-Ray date / result					
TBC test / date / result					

* Used by permission of the University of Florida Division of Intercollegiate Athletics.

7. Lower Extremities
   assymetry / atrophy

   Hamstrings
   Knocknee?   etc.

8. Knees   (1°-3°)
   Instability
   (MC / LC / AC / PC)

   Effusion / Rom

   Signif. History?

9. Feet / Ankles

10. Upper Extremities
    Rom, Atrophy, etc.
    History of dislocation
    or signif. trauma?

11. Spine

12. Neurological
    Gait / DTR, etc.

IT IS NEVER TOO EARLY OR TOO LATE!

That's right! Now may be just the right time to start this introduction to Athletic Training Course. Just a few hours a week of study can help your Student Trainers be stars of the team. Remember, there is another sports season just around the corner.

Every year several hundred student trainers are awarded scholarships and jobs as college and university student trainers. Nearly all of these have taken the Cramer Course. Start a new student trainer now.

Here is the 1972 application form for Cramer's "Extension Course in Athletic Training". It is prepared for officially appointed Student Trainers.

The cost will be $5.00 for each student, check forwarded with his application. Send to Cramer Student Trainer Course, Gardner, Kansas U.S.A. 66030

PLEASE TYPE OR PRINT THIS FORM

School _____ Date _____

Address _____ P.O. Box _____

City _____ State _____ Zip _____ Code _____ (Required)

Coach's Name _____

1972 STUDENT TRAINER COURSE APPLICATION FORM

Name _____

Address (Home) _____ R.R. _____ R.R. Box _____ P.O. Box _____

City _____ State _____ Zip _____ Code _____ (Required)

Age _____ Circle Year of High School Graduation

72 73 74 75 76

☐ $5.00 enclosed per Student

IN ORDER FOR STUDENT TO BE ENROLLED—ALL OF FORM MUST BE COMPLETED.

Send to: Cramer Student Trainer GARDNER, KANSAS U.S.A. 66030

ATHLETIC TRAINING IN THE SEVENTIES!

Here is the 1972 application form for Cramer's "Extension Course in Athletic Training". It is prepared for officially appointed student trainers.

Cramers regret that because of increased costs of printing, handling, and mailing, it is not possible to provide this course free. The cost will be $5.00 for each student, check forwarded with his application.

The course consists of a new book "Athletic Training in the Seventies", numerous lessons, charts, review questions, and practical work applications. It will be mailed complete to the coach making the appointment immediately upon receipt of the application. It is now felt since there is a charge that the coach should deliver the course to the student and help him get started right.

The coach making the appointment will be sent a set of review questions, certificate of accomplishment, and a student trainer emblem for presentation to the student trainer.

The student will need some supplies to carry out the practical work assignments. Most or all of these may be on hand in the training room. For the convenience of those students who do not have these items, Cramer's have available a special training supplies package for $6.75.

WHO ARE GOOD PROSPECTS?

1. Freshman and Sophomore high school students because: (a) interests formed early are often more lasting; and (b) the school will have the benefit of having several trainers with more experience by starting new younger ones each year.

2. A student with above average grades. It takes a lot of time to be a good trainer, and it is hardly fair to ask for this time from a student with serious academic problems.

3. A burning desire to be a part of athletics.

THERE IS COMPETITION IN GROUP STUDY

Coach, you may have several student trainers interested in taking the "Athletic Training in the Seventies!" course. Experience shows that many of these young people enjoy studying this subject together. Studying as a group has some advantages. There is a spirit of competition. Perhaps a testing program could be used to select the Head Student Trainer for that particular class. Also group study supplies the individual with someone he can practice on. It encourages regular study habits and continual progress as the class moves along together. Outside help might be encouraged to work more with a group than with an individual (example: team doctor, local professional trainer, etc.).

THIS IS BUDGET TIME !

This is it for many schools. Coach make sure you provide for coaching schools for the coaches and don't forget the student trainer clinics in your area. It is always an incentive to any student trainer to attend these one and two day study-work sessions. Check your training supplies—don't get caught short.

HOW TO DETERMINE A TRAINING ROOM BUDGET*

What Are Your Needs? What Is Your Budget?	Small Budget	Moderate Budget	Big Budget
Adhesive tape	X	X	X
Adhesive wall rack		X	X
Ankle wraps		X	X
Applicators (swab sticks)	X	X	X
Blankets		X	X
Braces (knees, etc.)			X
Bulletin Board			X
Cabinets (with lock)		X	X
Casting material		X	X
Chairs or benches		X	X
Clean walls and floors	X	X	X
Clippers (electric & blade)	X	X	X
Crutches	X	X	X
Cupboards for storage		X	X
Diathermy (shortwave)			X
Elastic adhesive tape		X	X
Eye cup	X	X	X
Felt (1/8", 1/4", 3/8", 1/2")	X	X	X
Fire extinguisher		X	X
Gauze (1/2", 1", 2", 3")	X	X	X
Heat lamp (infra red)	X	X	X
Heating System for Room		X	X

What Are Your Needs? What Is Your Budget?	Small Budget	Moderate Budget	Big Budget
Mats			X
Hanging bars		X	X
Resistance equipment			X
Shoulder wheel			X
Knee strengthener			X
Salt dispenser	X	X	X
Scales and weight chart	X	X	X
Scissors	X	X	X
Sink with hot water		X	X
Sheets		X	X
Slings	X	X	X
Steam cabinet			X
Steam room			X
Sterilizer		X	X
Sterile Pads (3x3, 4x4 gauze)	X	X	X
Stockinette		X	X
Stretcher	X	X	X
Sponge rubber (1/4", 1/2", 1", 2")	X	X	X
Splints	X	X	X
Surgical lamp (spotlight)			X
Table (training, taping)	X	X	X

* From Bike Catalog, The Kendall Company, Bike Sales Division, p. 9.

Heel Cups			X
Ice bag (Ice In Towel)		X	X
Lighting system and electrical outlets	X	X	X
Moleskin		X	X
Paraffin bath			X
Protective Equipment			
Anklet		X	X
Elbow		X	X
Face	X	X	X
Fracture glove		X	X
Forearm		X	X
Hand		X	X
Hip		X	X
Knee		X	X
Low Back		X	X
Mouthpiece	X	X	X
Ribs		X	X
Thigh		X	X
Wrist		X	
Refrigerator			X
Rehabilitation Room			X
Rehabilitation Equipment			X
Traction			X

Table for supplies	X	X	X
Tape cutters	X	X	X
Tape remover	X	X	X
Telephone			X
Thermometers	X	X	X
Toilet easily available			X
Tongue blades	X	X	X
Tourniquet	X	X	X
Toweling	X	X	X
Training table (portable)			X
Tweezers	X	X	X
Ventilating fan			X
Vibrator (hand)			X
Warbag (Trainer's Field Kit)	X	X	X
Wheel chair			X
Weights (training and rehabil.)		X	X
Whirlpool bath (varied sizes)		X	X
Miscellaneous frills			
Hair drier		X	X
Music piped in	X	X	X
Flashlight	X	X	X
Vibrating couch			X

Index